Blueprints Q&A
STEP 2: OBSTETRICS AND GYNECOLOGY

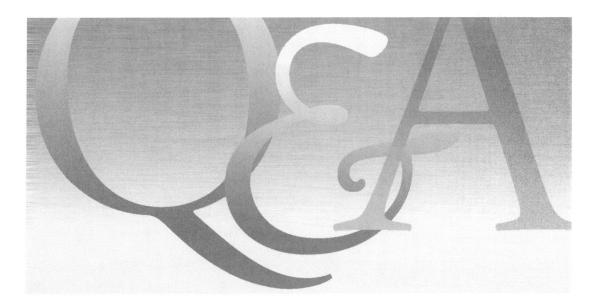

Blueprints Q&A
STEP 2: OBSTETRICS AND GYNECOLOGY

SERIES EDITOR:

Michael S. Clement, MD

Fellow, American Academy of Pediatrics
Mountain Park Health Center
Phoenix, Arizona
Clinical Lecturer in Family
   and Community Medicine
University of Arizona College of Medicine
Consultant, Arizona Department
   of Health Services

EDITOR:

James R. Mouer, MD

Clinical Associate Professor
University of Arizona College of Medicine
Associate Program Director
Phoenix Integrated Residency Program
   in Obstetrics and Gynecology
Medical Director, Department of
   Reproductive Medicine
Saint Joseph's Hospital
Phoenix, Arizona

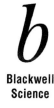

Blackwell
Science

EDITORIAL OFFICES:

Commerce Place, 350 Main Street,
Malden, Massachusetts 02148, USA

Osney Mead, Oxford OX2 0EL, England

25 John Street, London WC1N 2BS, England

23 Ainslie Place, Edinburgh EH3 6AJ, Scotland

54 University Street, Carlton, Victoria 3053, Australia

OTHER EDITORIAL OFFICES:

Blackwell Wissenschafts-Verlag GmbH,
Kurfürstendamm 57, 10707 Berlin, Germany

Blackwell Science KK, MG Kodenmacho Building,
7-10 Kodenmacho Nihombashi, Chuo-ku,
Tokyo 104, Japan

Iowa State University Press, A Blackwell Science Company,
2121 S. State Avenue, Ames, Iowa 50014-8300, USA

DISTRIBUTORS:

The Americas
Blackwell Publishing
c/o AIDC
P.O. Box 20
50 Winter Sport Lane
Williston, VT 05495-0020
(Telephone orders: 800-216-2522;
fax orders: 802-864-7626)

Australia Blackwell Science Pty, Ltd.
54 University Street
Carlton, Victoria 3053
(Telephone orders: 03-9347-0300;
fax orders: 03-9349-3016)

Outside The Americas and Australia
Blackwell Science, Ltd.
c/o Marston Book Services, Ltd., P.O. Box 269
Abingdon, Oxon OX14 4YN, England
(Telephone orders: 44-01235-465500;
fax orders: 44-01235-465555)

Acquisitions: Beverly Copland

Development: Angela Gagliano

Production: Irene Herlihy

Manufacturing: Lisa Flanagan

Marketing Manager: Toni Fournier

Cover design by Hannus Design

Typeset by Software Services

Printed and bound by Courier-Stoughton

Printed in the United States of America

01 02 03 04 5 4 3 2 1

The Blackwell Science logo is a trade mark of Blackwell Science Ltd., registered at the United Kingdom Trade Marks Registry

Library of Congress Cataloging-in-Publication Data

Blueprints Q & A step 2. Obstetrics and gynecology / editor, James R. Mouer.
    p. ; cm.—(Blueprints Q & A step 2 series)
  ISBN 0-632-04594-9 (pbk.)
  1. Gynecology—Examinations, questions, etc.
  2. Obstetrics—Examinations, questions, etc.
  3. Physicians—Licenses—United States—Study guides.
  [DNLM: 1. Genital Diseases, Female—Examination Questions. 2. Delivery—Examination Questions.
3. Pregnancy Complications—Examination Questions.
WP 18.2 B658 2002] I. Title: Blueprints Q&A step 2.
Obstetrics and gynecology. II. Title: Obstetrics and gynecology. III. Mouer, James R. IV. Series.
  RG111 .B58 2002
  618'.076—dc21   2001003188

Notice: The indications and dosages of all drugs in this book have been recommended in the medical literature and conform to the practices of the general community. The medications described and treatment prescriptions suggested do not necessarily have specific approval by the Food and Drug Administration for use in the diseases and dosages for which they are recommended. The package insert for each drug should be consulted for use and dosage as approved by the FDA. Because standards for usage change, it is advisable to keep abreast of revised recommendations, particularly those concerning new drugs.

CONTRIBUTORS:

Dean Coonrod, MD
Clinical Assistant Professor
University of Arizona College of Medicine
Phoenix, Arizona

Having attended Seattle Pacific University for undergraduate study, Dean then went on to the University of Eastern Washington Medical School to earn his medical degree. After receiving a Masters of Public Health in Epidemiology, he now specializes in Perinatal Epidemiology.

Glen Y. Kishi, MD
Assistant Professor of Clinical Obstetrics
University of Arizona College of Medicine
Phoenix, Arizona

After earning a BS in Chemical Engineering from the University of California, Davis, Glen then received his medical degree from the University of California, Irvine. Specializing in Medical Education, Glen has received numerous awards for excellence in teaching and education.

Beth Hamilton, MD
Resident in Obstetrics and Gynecology
Phoenix Integrated Residency Program
  in Obstetrics and Gynecology
Phoenix, Arizona

Beth attended the University of Southern California at Los Angeles for both her undergraduate and medical school study.

REVIEWERS:

Dominic Biney-Amissah, MD
Class of 2000
The University of Medicine and Dentistry
  of New Jersey—Robert Wood Johnson
  Medical School
Camden, New Jersey

Joseph Cassara, MD
Class of 2001
University of Vermont
Burlington, Vermont

Kenneth Galeckas, MD
Class of 2001
Boston University School of Medicine
Boston, Massachusetts

Jennifer Hale, MD
Class of 2001
University of Health Sciences—College
  of Osteopathic Medicine
Kansas City, Missouri

Brandon Johnson, MD
Class of 1999
University of Alabama School of Medicine
Birmingham, Alabama
Resident in Internal Medicine
Baptist Hospital
Birmingham, Alabama

PREFACE

The *Blueprints* Q&A Step 2 series has been developed to complement our core content *Blueprints* books. Each *Blueprints* Q&A Step 2 book (*Medicine, Pediatrics, Surgery, Psychiatry, and Obstetrics/Gynecology*) was written by residents seeking to provide fourth-year medical students with the highest quality of practice USMLE questions.

Each book covers a single discipline, allowing you to use them during both rotation exams as well as for review prior to Boards. For each book, 100 review questions are presented that cover content typical to the Step 2 USMLE. The questions are divided into two groups of 50 in order to simulate the length of one block of questions on the exam.

Answers are found at the end of each book, with the correct option screened. Accompanying the correct answer is a discussion of why the other options are incorrect. This allows for even the wrong answers to provide you with a valuable learning experience.

Blackwell has been fortunate to work with expert editors and residents—people like you who have studied for and passed the Boards. They sought to provide you with the very best practice prior to taking the Boards.

We welcome feedback and suggestions you may have about this book or any in the *Blueprints* series. Send to blue@blacksci.com.

All of the authors and staff at Blackwell wish you well on the Boards and in your medical future.

FIGURE CREDITS

The following figures were modified with permission from the Publisher.

Figure 2. Repke JT. Intrapartum Obstetrics. New York: Churchill Livingstone, 1996:80–81.

Figure 7. DeCherney A, Pernow M. Current Obstetrics and Gynecologic Diagnosis and Treatment. Norwalk, CT: Appleton & Lange, 1994:299.

Figure 9. DeCherney A, Pernow M. Current Obstetrics and Gynecologic Diagnosis and Treatment. Norwalk, CT: Appleton & Lange, 1994:299.

Figure 18. Gabbe SG, Niebyl JR, Simpson JL. Obstetrics: Normal and Problem Pregnancies. 2nd ed. New York: Churchill Livingstone, 1991:601.

Figure 20. Speroff L, Glass RH, Kase NG. Clinical Gynecologic Endocrinology and Infertility. 5th ed. Baltimore: Williams & Wilkins, 1994:378.

Figure 41. Beckman CC, Ling F. Obstetrics and Gynecology for Medical Students. Baltimore: Williams & Wilkins, 1992:398.

Figure 42. Speroff L, Darney PA. A Clinical Guide for Contraception. 2nd ed. Baltimore: Williams & Wilkins, 1996:680.

Figure 47. Speroff L, Darney PA. A Clinical Guide for Contraception. 2nd ed. Baltimore: Williams & Wilkins, 1996:247.

Figure 52. Callahan TL, Caughey AB, Heffner LJ. Blueprints in Obstetrics and Gynecology. 2nd ed. Malden, MA: Blackwell Science, 2001:12.

Figure 57. Callahan TL, Caughey AB, Heffner LJ. Blueprints in Obstetrics and Gynecology. 2nd ed. Malden, MA: Blackwell Science, 2001:120.

Figure 59. Champion RH. Textbook of Dermatology. 5th ed. Oxford: Blackwell Science, 1992:2852.

Figure 70. Crissey JT. Manual of Medical Mycology. Boston: Blackwell Science, 1995:90.

Figure 72. Beckman CC, et al. Obstetrics and Gynecology for Medical Students. 2nd ed. Baltimore: Williams & Wilkins, 1995:176.

Figure 83. Benson RC, Pernoll ML. Handbook of Obstetrics and Gynecology. 9th ed. New York: McGraw-Hill, 1994:157.

Figure 87. Szulman AE, J Reprod Med 1985, 29:288.

Figure 88. Blackwell RE. Women's Medicine. 1996:317.

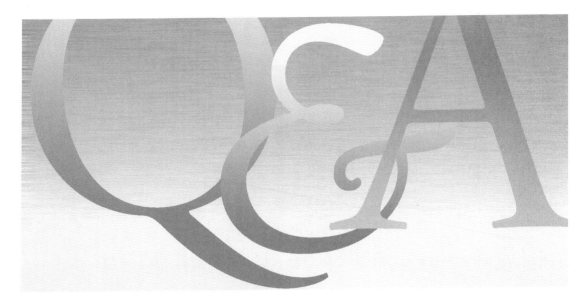

BLOCK **ONE**

QUESTIONS

QUESTION 1

A 28-year-old secundigravida at 40 weeks' gestation is undergoing a trial of labor. Her prior delivery was complicated by cephalopelvic disproportion and required a low transverse cesarean section for delivery. For the last 4 hours, she has been on pitocin for augmentation of her contractions. About 30 minutes ago she started complaining of persistent lower abdominal pain. Repetitive variable decelerations began at the same time. Your exam of the patient notes that she is 3 cm dilated, has moderate vaginal bleeding, and the presenting part is no longer palpable. What is the most likely diagnosis?

A. Placental abruption

B. Placenta previa

C. Uterine hyperstimulation

D. Uterine rupture

E. Cord prolapse

QUESTION 2

A 21-year-old nulliparous woman is in active labor. Her membranes have been ruptured for the last 4 hours. She is having contractions every 3–5 minutes, each lasting about 60 seconds and of moderate intensity. In your evaluation of her progress, you perform a cervical exam and note that she is 5 cm dilated. The fetal vertex and skull sutures are readily palpable. You determine that the current position of the fetal vertex (see Figure 2D) is:

A. Occiput anterior

B. Right occiput anterior

C. Left occiput anterior

D. Right occiput posterior

E. Left occiput posterior

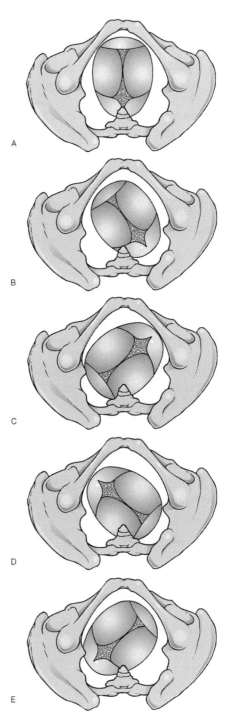

A

B

C

D

E

FIGURE 2

QUESTION 3

A 20-year-old multiparous woman underwent AFP testing at 16 weeks' gestation. The initial result was 0.3 multiple of the median (MoM) (normal 0.5–2.0 MoM). The result of a repeat test performed 5 days later was 0.2 multiple of the median. The abnormality most likely to be associated with these results is:

A. Trisomy 21

B. Triploidy

C. Twin pregnancy

D. Meningomyelocele

E. Trisomy 13

QUESTION 4

A woman at 32 weeks' gestation is brought to the emergency room following an automobile accident. She has no obvious head injury. Her temperature is 36.7°C (98°F), pulse 110, and BP 80/50. Her skin is cool and clammy. The lower portion of her abdomen is tense and tender. Bowel sounds are decreased and the fetal heart tones are absent. The most likely diagnosis is:

A. Ruptured spleen

B. Ruptured uterus

C. Perforated viscus

D. Abruptio placentae

E. Ruptured bladder

QUESTION 5

A 20-year-old primigravid comes to you for her first prenatal visit at 12 weeks. She works in a daycare facility and developed a maculopapular rash at 11 weeks' gestation. It disappears after 3 days and she feels fine.

A. You should reassure her since the symptoms were mild.

B. Offer termination of the pregnancy.

C. Obtain her rubella IgG titer.

D. Obtain a throat culture and treat with penicillin for 10 days.

E. Obtain a toxoplasmosis IgG titer.

QUESTION 6

The most reliable diagnostic finding associated with chorioamnionitis is:

A. Maternal leukocytosis

B. Maternal tachycardia

C. Uterine tenderness

D. Maternal fever

E. Maternal bacteremia

QUESTION 7

A 23-year-old multipara has been in active labor for the last 8 hours. Her cervix is dilated to 8 cm and the fetal vertex is at plus 2 station. The fetus is of average size and she has had a prior uneventful 9-pound fetus deliver vaginally. Recently, her contractions have been augmented by an oxytocin intravenous infusion. Membranes are ruptured and the amniotic fluid is clear. The patient is afebrile and normotensive. She has not required any medication for pain control. Her nurse has notified you of a recent change in the character of the fetal heart tracing. On arrival at the patient's bedside, you note the following fetal heart tracing. Of the following, which is the most appropriate next step:

A. Immediate forceps delivery

B. Immediate cesarean delivery

C. Amnioinfusion of the fetus and supplemental oxygen to the mother

D. Discontinue oxytocin infusion and give supplemental oxygen to the mother.

E. Observation and reevaluation in 2 hours

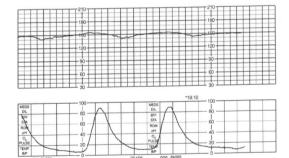

FIGURE 7

QUESTION 8

At 32 weeks' EGA, a 26-year-old multipara has been hospitalized for 10 days for PROM. She had a previous LTCS because of arrested dilation. For 2 hours she has had light vaginal bleeding and contractions every 15 minutes. Over the past 30 minutes the bleeding has increased slightly, and she experiences lower abdominal pain between contractions. Her temperature is 37.0°C (98.6°F). The uterus is tender and the FHR is 170. Platelet count is 130K, leukocyte count is 14.3K, serum fibrinogen is 225 mg/dl, and the assay for fibrin split products is positive. Which of the following is the most likely diagnosis?

A. Complete placenta previa

B. Chorioamnionitis

C. Abruptio placentae

D. Uterine scar dehiscence

E. HELLP syndrome

QUESTION 9

A 28-year-old nulligravid has been in active labor for the last 4 hours. Her labor was induced with an oxytocin intravenous infusion. Her cervix is dilated to 6 cm, and the fetal vertex is at plus 1 station. You estimate the fetus to weigh approximately 7 pounds, and by clinical exam you have determined that the maternal pelvis is adequate. Membranes are ruptured and the amniotic fluid is clear. The patient is afebrile and normotensive. She has not required any medication for pain control. Her nurse has notified you of a recent change in the character of the fetal heart tracing. On arrival at the patient's bedside, you note the following fetal heart tracing. Of the following, which is the most appropriate next step?

A. Immediate forceps delivery

B. Immediate cesarean delivery

C. Amnioinfusion of the fetus and supplemental oxygen to the mother

D. Discontinue oxytocin infusion and give supplemental oxygen to the mother.

E. Observation and reevaluation in 2 hours

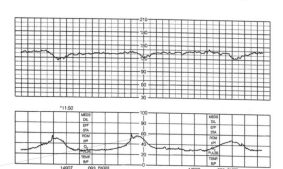

FIGURE 9

QUESTION 10

A patient at 28 weeks' EGA was hospitalized recently with preterm labor. Contractions ceased after parenteral tocolysis, and she was placed on 2.5 mg of oral terbutaline every 4 hours. When she is seen on rounds the following morning, she is asymptomatic, her lungs are clear to auscultation, and she denies uterine contractions. Pulse rate is 110 bpm and regular. A II/VI systolic murmur is noted along the left sternal border. The next appropriate step in the management of this patient is to:

A. Decrease the dose.

B. Discontinue the tocolytic agent.

C. Continue present management.

D. Obtain an electrocardiogram (ECG).

E. Lengthen the interval between doses.

QUESTION 11

You are asked to consult on a laboring 29-year-old multipara in active labor. The patient is concerned about the large size of her fetus. She is concerned about the possibility of this fetus having a difficult delivery. She tells you that her last delivery was complicated by a shoulder dystocia. You tell her that shoulder dystocia has been associated with all of the following EXCEPT:

A. Previous shoulder dystocia

B. Maternal obesity

C. Paternal diabetes

D. Prolonged second stage of labor

E. Fetal macrosomia

QUESTION 12

You are asked to consult on a young woman with a preexisting cardiac defect. She wants to become pregnant in the near future and seeks advice about what risks to her health that this will create. You tell that the highest maternal mortality rates are associated with which of the following cardiac defects:

A. Aortic stenosis

B. Mitral stenosis

C. Ebstein anomaly

D. Atrial-septal defect

E. Eisenmenger syndrome

QUESTION 13

A 32-year-old woman at 21 weeks' gestation presents with acute shortness of breath and pleuritic chest pain. Her medical history is significant for antiphospholipid antibody syndrome. Which of the following tests would be most helpful in confirming the diagnosis?

A. Chest radiograph

B. Electrocardiogram

C. Ventilation perfusion scan

D. Lower extremity venous doppler

E. Arterial blood gas

QUESTION 14

Which of the following antibodies is most likely to cause hemolytic disease in a neonate?

A. Anti Kell

B. Anti E

C. Anti M

D. Anti Lewis

E. Anti P

QUESTION 15

A 25-year-old woman, gravida 2, para 1, with chronic hypertension, is at 38 weeks' gestation. Ultrasound examination shows an amniotic fluid index of 4 cm and an estimated fetal weight below the 10th percentile. A nonstress test (NST) is nonreactive with absent variability, and a subsequent contraction stress test (CST) is positive. Her Bishop score is 4. Which of the following should be the next step in managing this patient?

A. Cordocentesis for fetal karyotype

B. Cordocentesis for fetal blood pH

C. Biophysical profile

D. Immediate delivery

E. Repeat contraction stress test in 1 week

QUESTION 16

A 25-year-old multiparous patient at 28 weeks' gestation has condyloma lata. Six hours after receiving her first intramuscular dose of penicillin G benzathine, 2.4 mIU, she experiences fever, chills, malaise, headache, and myalgia. She also states that her lesions have become acutely painful. Her temperature is 38.3°C (100.9°F), pulse is 110 bpm, blood pressure in 90/60 mm Hg, and respirations are 24/min. The most likely diagnosis is

A. Waterhouse–Friderichsen syndrome

B. Allergic reaction to penicillin

C. Jarisch–Herxheimer reaction

D. Secondary bacteremia

E. Disseminated HPV viremia

QUESTION 17

If the embryonic disc divides 14 days after fertilization, the result is a:

A. Diamniotic, dichorionic placentation

B. Diamniotic, monochorionic placentation

C. Velamentous cord insertion

D. Conjoined twins

E. Acardia

QUESTION 18

A multipara has just delivered a 10-pound infant after a precipitous labor. When the placenta delivers a short while later, it appears to be attached to a large round firm mass that fills the vagina. A large amount of active bright red vaginal bleeding is noted. The patient becomes pale and her blood pressure is noted to be 70/30 mm Hg. What is the most likely diagnosis?

A. Intraabdominal hemorrhage

B. Uterine inversion

C. Retroperitoneal hemorrhage

D. Uterine atony

E. Uterine rupture

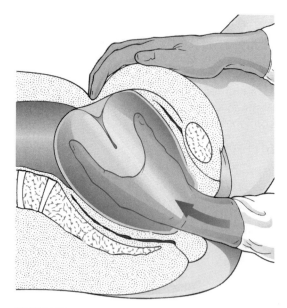

FIGURE 18

QUESTION 19

In order to stop intractable uterine bleeding from postpartum hemorrhage, ligation of the internal iliac arteries is performed. Blood flow will be greatly diminished in all of the following arteries EXCEPT:

A. Obturator

B. Superior gluteal

C. Inferior gluteal

D. Superior vesical

E. Superior rectal

QUESTION 20

During your yearly exam of a 13-year-old girl, you evaluate her pubertal development. Breast development started about 2 years ago, followed more recently by pubic and axillary hair growth. When you examine her from the side, you see the following breast contour (Figure 20D). This is an example of Tanner stage:

A. One

B. Two

C. Three

D. Four

E. Five

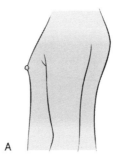
A

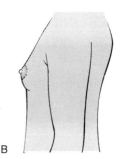
B

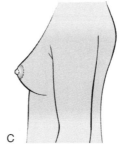
C

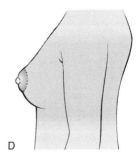
D

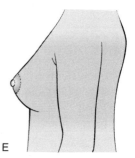
E

FIGURE 20

QUESTION 21

In utero, the highest concentration of oxygen is found in which of the following fetal vessels?

A. Abdominal aorta

B. Umbilical vein

C. Umbilical artery

D. Pulmonary artery

E. Femoral artery

QUESTION 22

Above the arcuate line, the fascia of what muscle lies adjacent to the peritoneum?

A. Pyramidalis

B. Rectus abdominus

C. External oblique

D. Internal oblique

E. Transversus abdominus

QUESTION 23

When evaluating the results of a human chorionic gonadotropin level in the maternal blood, the peak value occurs at which menstrual week of the pregnancy?

A. 3–4

B. 9–10

C. 14–16

D. 24–28

E. 36–42

QUESTION 24

In performing preconceptual counseling to a young couple, you inform them that the most susceptible time period for teratogen exposure to the human embryo is at which embryonic week (week after conception)?

A. 2 weeks

B. 6 weeks

C. 10 weeks

D. 14 weeks

E. 18 weeks

QUESTION 25

You are asked to see a young woman in the emergency department for a miscarriage. On exam, she has passed the conceptus, and no products of conception remain inside the uterus. The cervical os is closed and has minimal bleeding. Vital signs are stable. The patient is inquiring as to the reason for her miscarriage. Knowing that the most likely cause of this spontaneous abortion is due to aneuploidy, you can tell her that the most common chromosomal abnormality is:

A. Tetraploidy

B. Triploidy

C. Autosomal trisomy

D. Haploid of paternal origin

E. Diploid of paternal origin

QUESTION 26

A 36-year-old gravida 4 para 4 presents to your office due to irregular vaginal bleeding. Her last delivery was 2 years ago and uncomplicated. Since then, she has had two normal periods, but only intermittent spotting and bleeding for the last 7 months. Pelvic exam demonstrates a normal sized uterus and adnexa. You perform an endometrial biopsy to rule out the possibility of a malignancy. The biopsy finding is most likely to show:

A. Endometrial adenocarcinoma

B. Adenomatous hyperplasia with atypia

C. Adenomatous hyperplasia without atypia

D. Proliferative endometrium

E. Arias Stella reaction

QUESTION 27

A 15-year-old patient requests evaluation of masculinization and failure to begin menstruation. She was taller than her peers during childhood. Pubic hair growth began at 6 years, excessive facial hair growth began at 10. She now shaves 3–4 times a week. She is 150 cm (63 inches) tall, and her BP is 120/80. She has prominent musculature, and her breasts are Tanner stage 2. Pelvic exam reveals an enlarged clitoris, moderate posterior labial-scrotal fusion, and a cervix in the vaginal vault. There are no pelvic masses on bimanual exam. This patient's sex chromosomes are most likely:

A. XX

B. XXY

C. X/XY

D. XX/XY

E. XYY

QUESTION 28

A concerned mother brings in her 16-year-old daughter because she hasn't ever had a menstrual period. On exam, the girl is 5 feet 8 inches tall with mature adult breast development and scant to no pubic nor axillary hair. Vaginal exam is difficult and you are unable to identify a cervix nor palpate a uterus. The most likely diagnosis is:

A. Androgenital syndrome

B. Imperforate hymen

C. Turner syndrome

D. Complete androgen insensitivity syndrome

E. Rokitansky Kuster Hauser syndrome

QUESTION 29

A 27-year-old patient complains of 6 months of amenorrhea. A pregnancy test is negative. Which of the following is the most likely cause of secondary amenorrhea in this patient?

A. Abnormal chromosomes

B. Asherman syndrome

C. Hypothyroidism

D. Prolactinoma

E. Anovulation

QUESTION 30

A 27-year-old sexually active woman presents to your office for evaluation. She hasn't had her period for the last 3 months. Prior to that time, they were regular, every 28 days, with a light flow lasting for 4 days. In your initial evaluation of her condition, which of the following serum tests is most important?

A. Prolactin

B. Luteinizing hormone (LH)

C. Estimated free thyroxine

D. Human chorionic gonadotropin (hCG)

E. Follicle stimulating hormone (FSH)

QUESTION 31

A 14-year-old girl is brought in by her mother for monthly cyclic pelvic pain. She has never had a menstrual period. At age 10 she began developing breasts followed several months later by pubic hair. She is 5 feet 7 inches tall. Currently she has Tanner stage 4 breasts and Tanner stage 4 pubic hair. On perineal exam you see a suburethral bluish bulge. Rectal exam notes a midline fullness. The most likely diagnosis is:

A. Transverse vaginal septum

B. Imperforate hymen

C. Gonadal dysgenesis

D. Complete androgen insensitivity syndrome

E. Congenital adrenal hyperplasia

QUESTION 32

A 21-year-old primigravida has just given birth. Examining her infant, you note that it has what appears to be an enlarged protuberant clitoris along with partially fused, rugated, and pigmented labia majora. No palpable gonads are noted. Which of the following enzyme defects is the infant most likely to have?

A. 11 beta hydroxylase

B. 3 beta hydroxysteroid dehydrogenase

C. 17 beta hydroxysteroid dehydrogenase

D. 21 alpha hydroxylase

E. 17,20 desmolase

QUESTION 33

In evaluating a reproductive age woman who presents with amenorrhea, which of the following conditions will result in a positive (withdrawal) progesterone challenge test?

A. Pregnancy

B. Ovarian failure

C. Pituitary failure

D. Mullerian agenesis

E. Polycystic ovary (PCO) syndrome

QUESTION 34

A young couple undergo a postcoital test as part of an infertility evaluation. Several hours after coitus, the cervical mucus is thick and tenacious. No sperm are seen in the mucus, although they are present in the vagina. Semen analysis is normal. Eight days later, the patient menstruates. Her basal body temperature (BBT) record for that cycle indicates ovulation and a normal luteal phase. The most appropriate management of this patient is to:

A. Perform antisperm antibody studies.

B. Attempt intrauterine insemination with washed sperm.

C. Prescribe low dose estrogen for days 7–14 of the cycle.

D. Repeat the postcoital test 6–7 days earlier in the next cycle.

E. Start clomiphene citrate therapy on days 5–9 of the cycle.

QUESTION 35

For the last 5 years, this obese 33-year-old nulligravid has been unsuccessful in her attempts at getting pregnant. Her menses are irregular and have been that way since menarche at age 12. She has never used contraception. She frequently has to shave unsightly facial hair. Her pelvic exam shows thin watery cervical mucus, with somewhat enlarged adnexa bilaterally. All of the following would be helpful in the workup and/or management of this condition EXCEPT:

A. Serum fasting glucose to insulin ratio

B. Serum free testosterone level

C. Serum estradiol level

D. Endometrial biopsy

E. Ovulation induction with clomiphene citrate

QUESTION 36

A 35-year-old woman presents to your office. She and her 32-year-old husband have been unsuccessful in their attempts to get pregnant for the last 6 years. He has fathered two children in a prior marriage and has a normal semen analysis. Her basal body temperature chart is biphasic. Her past history notes multiple episodes of chlamydia and gonorrhea. A hysterosalpingogram demonstrates blocked fallopian tubes bilaterally, and a laparoscope notes dense and profuse peritubal and pelvic adhesions, along with bilateral clubbed tubes. The most appropriate fertility treatment would be:

A. Intrauterine insemination with husband's sperm (IUI)

B. Intracytoplasmic sperm injection with husband's sperm (ICSI)

C. Gonadotropin induction of ovulation

D. In vitro fertilization (IVF)

E. Gamete intrafallopian transfer (GIFT)

QUESTION 37

During the midluteal phase, progesterone secretion occurs immediately after pulsatile secretion of:

A. Follicle stimulating hormone (FSH)

B. Luteinizing hormone (LH)

C. Estradiol

D. Inhibin

E. Activin

QUESTION 38

Estrogen replacement therapy in postmeno-pausal women has been shown to do all of the following EXCEPT:

A. Reduce the risk of osteoporosis.

B. Reduce the risk of coronary heart disease.

C. Reduce the risk of ovarian cancer.

D. Reduce the risk of bowel cancer.

E. Prevent genitourinary atrophy.

QUESTION 39

In normal pubertal development, which of the following is true?

A. Pubarche usually precedes thelarche.

B. Menarche usually precedes pubarche.

C. Menarche usually precedes peak height growth velocity.

D. Regular ovulatory cycles occur about 2 years after menarche.

E. Ovulation must occur before menses can begin.

QUESTION 40

A 16-year-old girl presents to your office for gyne-cologic evaluation. She has never had any vagi-nal bleeding. She does not recall ever having started her breast development, nor has she had any growth of axillary or pubic hair. Her height is 59 inches. On routine physical exam you see cubi-tus valgus of the elbows, excess skin of the neck, and a shield-shaped chest with wide-spaced nip-ples. What is the most appropriate next step in her evaluation?

A. Hormone replacement therapy

B. Growth hormone therapy

C. Estradiol serum level

D. Pelvic ultrasonography

E. Gonadotropin levels

QUESTION 41

The following statements are true about uterine leiomyomas EXCEPT:

A. They are 5 times more common in African-American women when compared to Caucasian women.

B. They can be diagnosed by ultrasound.

C. They have been associated with infertility.

D. They can be suppressed by estrogen therapy.

E. They are asymptomatic in over 50% of those who have them.

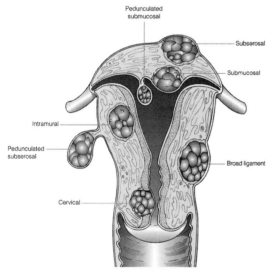

FIGURE 41

QUESTION 42

The main contraceptive action of the copper-based intrauterine device is:

A. Prevention of implantation of the fertilized ovum

B. Cessation of ovulation

C. Induced abortion

D. Production of a spermicidal environment

E. Elevation of serum copper level

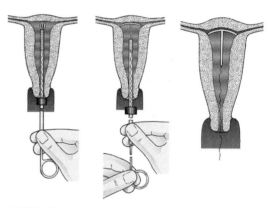

FIGURE 42

QUESTION 43

Of the following forms of contraception, women using which of the following have the highest rate of ectopic pregnancy?

A. No contraception

B. Diaphragm

C. Oral contraceptive pills

D. Injectable progestin (depo provera)

E. Intrauterine device

QUESTION 44

You are asked to see a young woman in the Emergency Department after an alleged sexual assault that occurred today. She is an otherwise healthy 28 years old. A serum pregnancy test is negative. Her menstrual cycle is regular, every 28 days, and her last period was 14 days ago. She is not currently on contraception and desires to minimize her chance of becoming pregnant from this episode. Of the following, the best option is:

A. Immediate placement of a copper bearing intrauterine device

B. Give Ovral 2 tablets followed by two more tablets 12 hours later.

C. Start a daily low dose triphasic birth control pill.

D. Start diethylstilbestrol (DES) 50 mg per day for 5 days.

E. Immediate dilation and suction curettage

QUESTION 45

A 28-year-old G2P2 woman, whose LMP began yesterday, noticed a painful mass in her left breast. Examination discloses a discrete 2 cm apparently cystic mass in the upper outer quadrant. Supra-clavicular and axillary areas are negative. The most appropriate next step in management is:

A. Mammography

B. Excisional biopsy

C. Needle aspiration

D. Reexamination after onset of menses

E. Excisional biopsy with lymph node sampling

QUESTION 46

The most frequent cause of dyspareunia is:

A. Vaginismus

B. Endometriosis

C. Retroverted uterus

D. Inadequate vaginal lubrication

E. Pelvic inflammatory disease

QUESTION 47

A 21-year-old sexually active woman comes to your office requesting a cervical cap for contraception. You advise her that the maximum number of hours that the cervical cap should be left in place is:

A. 4 hours

B. 12 hours

C. 24 hours

D. 36 hours

E. 48 hours

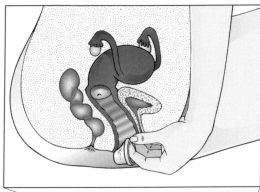

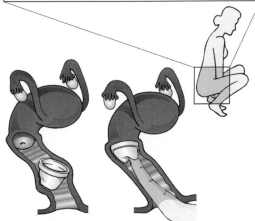

FIGURE 47

QUESTION 48

A 37-year-old woman, who complains of heavy painful menses, requests contraception. She smokes a pack of cigarettes a day. Of the following, the best choice of contraceptive for this patient is:

A. Copper t380a intrauterine device (IUD)

B. Low-dose, combined oral contraceptives

C. Contraceptive implant (Norplant)

D. Endometrial ablation

E. Hysterectomy

QUESTION 49

A healthy 40-year-old woman requests oral contraceptives. As her sole health care provider, appropriate evaluation includes all of the following tests EXCEPT:

A. Mammography

B. Pap test

C. Endometrial sampling

D. Blood lipid determination

E. Blood pressure determination

QUESTION 50

A 40-year-old multiparous patient presents with a 10-day history of heavy vaginal bleeding and lower abdominal cramping that began at the expected time of her menses. Pelvic examination reveals a 6-cm mass judged to be a prolapsed submucosal myoma protruding from the cervix on a 1.5-cm stalk. The uterus is enlarged to twice normal size and is mobile. Active bleeding is present, and the patient's hematocrit is 26%. Which of the following is optimal management at this time?

A. Transfusion and vaginal hysterectomy

B. Transfusion and abdominal hysterectomy

C. Biopsy of the mass and transfusion if necessary

D. Transvaginal myomectomy and transfusion if necessary

E. High dose birth control pills

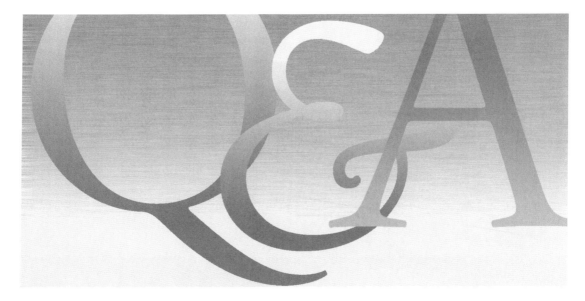

BLOCK **TWO**

QUESTIONS

QUESTION 51

A 13-year-old patient has had regular menses for 1 year, with debilitating pain beginning in the lower abdomen a few hours before menses and lasting 24 hours. Physical examination is completely normal. Optimal management at this time is:

A. Psychiatric referral

B. Diagnostic laparoscopy

C. Trial of oral contraceptives

D. Trial of prostaglandin synthetase inhibitors

E. Reassurance with follow-up evaluation in 6 months

QUESTION 52

A 16-year-old woman presents to the emergency department complaining of severe left-sided pelvic pain and vaginal spotting. Her last menstrual period was 6 weeks ago. A quantitative beta HCG is 9,000 mIU/ml. An endovaginal ultrasound notes a complex left adnexal mass, moderate free fluid, and no evidence of an intrauterine sac. The most likely site of this pregnancy is:

A. Cervix

B. Uterine cornua

C. Isthmus of the fallopian tube

D. Ampulla of the fallopian tube

E. Fimbria of the fallopian tube

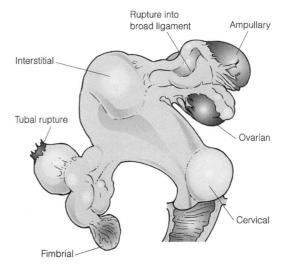

FIGURE 52

QUESTION 53

A 23-year-old sexually active woman with a prior history of pelvic inflammatory disease presents with sudden onset of pelvic pain. On initial workup and exam, you note the following: Beta HCG titer 5,400 mIU/ml; WBC 4,500 (units); differential: 63 PMNs, 0 Bands, 37 lymphocytes; temperature 37.3°C (99.1°F). An endovaginal ultrasound shows nothing in the uterus, a 2-cm simple left ovarian cyst, and moderate free fluid in the cul-de-sac. The most likely diagnosis is:

A. Recurrent pelvic inflammatory disease

B. Ectopic pregnancy

C. Ruptured ovarian cyst

D. Endometriosis

E. Irritable bowel syndrome

QUESTION 54

When taking a patient history, which of the following questions will most accurately ascertain the length of the patient's menstrual cycle?

A. How often do you menstruate?

B. Do you menstruate every month?

C. How many days are there between your periods?

D. How many days are there from the beginning of one period to the beginning of the next?

E. How many days are there from the end of one period to the beginning of the next?

QUESTION 55

Mixing vaginal discharge with potassium hydroxide (KOH) creates an odor that is helpful in diagnosing:

A. Bacterial vaginosis

B. Trichomoniasis

C. Moniliasis

D. Gonorrhea

E. Chlamydia

QUESTION 56

Of the following, which is the most appropriate initial antibiotic treatment for a tuboovarian abscess?

A. Clindamycin and ampicillin

B. Tetracycline and penicillin

C. Clindamycin and gentamicin

D. Ciprofloxacin and gentamicin

E. Ampicillin and gentamicin

QUESTION 57

A 23-year-old woman presents to your office complaining of several nontender, asymptomatic, slightly umbilicated, 3-mm nodules on her lower abdomen. Hypodermic probe of a nodule reveals a cheesy substance. Which of the following is the most likely diagnosis?

A. Sebaceous cysts

B. Condylomata lata

C. Lichen planus

D. Psoriasis

E. Molluscum contagiosum

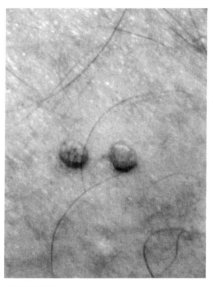

FIGURE 57

QUESTION 58

Pelvic inflammatory disease is characterized by all of the following EXCEPT:

A. Leukocytosis

B. Pelvic pain

C. Fever

D. Anemia

E. Cervical motion tenderness

QUESTION 59

A nonpregnant 17-year-old girl presents to your office for routine examination. On pelvic exam, you note several raised fleshy lesions on her vulva and vaginal wall. No vaginal nor cervical discharge is noted. Her inguinal nodes are slightly tender and palpable bilaterally. She appears to have a generalized maculopapular rash. On further questioning, she recollected a painless labial ulcer that resolved about 2 months ago. The best treatment regimen for this patient is:

A. Laser ablation of the vulvar and vaginal lesions

B. Trichloroacetic acid application of the vulvar and vaginal lesions

C. Benzathine penicillin g 2.4 million units IM, one dose

D. Benzathine penicillin g 2.4 million units IM, q week times three total doses

E. Acyclovir 400 mg po, 5 times per day for 14 days

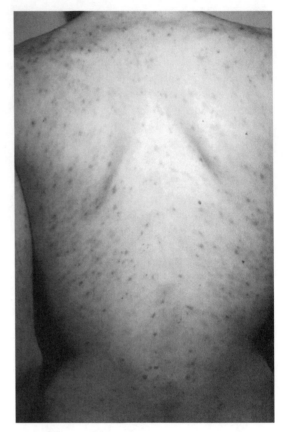

FIGURE 59

QUESTION 60

Three days after her menses started, this 21-year-old woman began having sudden onset of nausea, vomiting, diarrhea, and a flu-like malaise. She does not use tampons, but has had sexual relations in the last several days and uses a cervical cap for contraception. On evaluation, you find her blood pressure to be 75/35 mm Hg, pulse of 130 bpm, and an oral temperature of 39.3°C (102.7°F). She has a diffuse macular rash over her entire body. Of the following, which is correct?

A. Blood cultures will be positive for *Staphylococcus aureus*.

B. Blood cultures will be positive for *Neisseria gonorrhoeae*.

C. Most of the clinical signs and symptoms are due to a bacterial endotoxin.

D. Intravenous fluid resuscitation to correct hypotension is the first priority in therapy.

E. Beta lactamase resistant penicillin antibiotic therapy is the first priority in therapy.

QUESTION 61

A 20-year-old patient has urinary frequency and dysuria. Pelvic examination reveals a yellow discharge at the cervix and mild adnexal tenderness. The best immediate test to aid your diagnosis is:

A. Gram stain of a cervical smear

B. Peripheral leukocyte count

C. Cervical smear for *Chlamydia trachomatis*

D. Cervical culture on Thayer Martin medium

E. Dipstick urinalysis of specimen obtained by bladder catheterization

QUESTION 62

A 52-year-old woman presents to your office complaining of vaginal bleeding. Her last bleeding episode was 2 years ago. She is not on hormone replacement therapy. Her hemoglobin is 13.4. A vaginal ultrasound shows her uterus and adnexa to be normal size and an endometrial stripe of 11 mm. The next step in her evaluation should be:

A. Hysterectomy

B. Dilation and curettage

C. Endometrial biopsy

D. Endometrial ablation

E. Intermittent progestin therapy

QUESTION 63

At the time of her annual examination, you find an 11-week-sized irregular uterus on an asymptomatic 40-year-old woman. Her last exam 1 year prior was normal. Your next step in the management of this patient is:

A. Hysterectomy

B. Endometrial biopsy

C. Reexamination in 6 months

D. Fractional dilation and curettage

E. Gonadotropin releasing hormone agonist therapy

QUESTION 64

A 19-year-old nulligravid healthy woman comes to see you for her annual Pap smear and routine health care maintenance. During your routine pelvic exam, you note that she has a 5-cm cystic, nontender, mobile mass in her left adnexa. Rectovaginal exam confirms this and does not note any abnormalities in the cul-de-sac. Which of the following is the most appropriate next step?

A. Laparotomy with ovarian cystectomy

B. Repeat pelvic exam in 2 months

C. MRI scan of the pelvis

D. Ultrasound of the pelvis

E. Laparoscopy with ovarian cystectomy

QUESTION 65

A 22-year-old woman comes to the emergency department complaining of sudden onset of severe cramping in the right lower quadrant. Her temperature is 37.4°C (99.4°F), pulse is 90 bpm, and blood pressure is 100/70 mm Hg. The abdomen is tender to palpation in the right lower quadrant, and peritoneal signs are present. Pelvic examination reveals an exquisitely tender 8-cm right adnexal mass. Urine pregnancy test is negative. She continues to complain of unbearable pain. The most likely diagnosis is:

A. Appendicitis

B. Torsion of ovary

C. Ectopic pregnancy

D. Rupture of corpus luteum

E. Rupture of tuboovarian abscess

QUESTION 66

You are asked to evaluate a 6-year-old girl who has fallen off her brother's bicycle and is complaining of severe vulvar pain. The girl will not permit anyone to touch her vulva. However, on inspection, the upper labia majus is blue and there is vaginal bleeding. What is the next step in managing her injury?

A. Perform the examination under anesthesia.

B. Have her mother restrain her during the examination.

C. Have a medical assistant restrain her during the examination.

D. Send her home to use ice packs and reschedule the examination for the next day.

E. Perform a laparotomy to evaluate for penetrating trauma.

QUESTION 67

A 45-year-old otherwise healthy woman complains of urine loss with coughing, laughing, and sneezing. This has become noticeable since the vaginal delivery of her third child. Due to the urine loss, she finds it necessary to wear a pad when exercising or walking. On exam, you note a large midline bulge in the anterior vaginal wall that descends to the introitus on valsalva. The most likely reason for urine loss is:

A. Stress incontinence

B. Urge incontinence

C. Vesicovaginal fistula

D. Detrussor dyssynergia

E. Neurogenic bladder

QUESTION 68

During pregnancy, lactation is suppressed by the action of:

A. Insulin

B. Estrogen

C. Thyroid hormone (T4)

D. Human placental lactogen

E. Inhibin

QUESTION 69

A healthy 30-year-old primigravid woman at 16 weeks' gestation presents for prenatal care. She tells you that her biological brother has cystic fibrosis, and that their parents have no evidence of the disease. The father of the baby has no family history of cystic fibrosis. If the carrier rate in the general population is 1/22, what is the risk that this fetus will have cystic fibrosis?

A. 1/176

B. 1/132

C. 1/44

D. 1/66

E. 1/88

QUESTION 70

A 21-year-old woman at 24 weeks' gestation complains of severe vulvar itching and a grayish foul-smelling vaginal discharge. A saline wet mount slide shows the following on microscopic exam. The most likely diagnosis is:

A. *Candida albicans*

B. Bacterial vaginosis

C. Trichomoniasis

D. *Chlamydia trachomatis*

E. Human papilloma virus

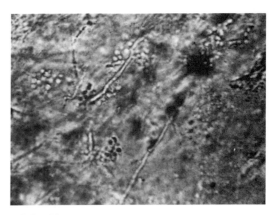

FIGURE 70

QUESTION 71

A female medical student at 10 weeks' gestation is starting an intravenous line in a patient who is a chronic active hepatitis B carrier. After placing the line, the student inadvertently sticks herself with the bloody needle. The student has never been immunized against hepatitis B and is susceptible. Which of the following is the best choice in managing her situation?

A. Immune globulin only

B. Hepatitis B vaccine only

C. Hepatitis B immune globulin only

D. Hepatitis B vaccine and hepatitis B immune globulin

E. Observation only

QUESTION 72

Engagement of the fetal head is defined by:

A. The leading edge of the fetal head is at the ischial spines.

B. The biparietal diameter is through the pelvic inlet.

C. The occipitofrontal diameter is through the pelvic inlet.

D. The lowest part of the head is at a plane between the ischial spines.

E. The leading edge of the fetal head is at the vaginal introitus.

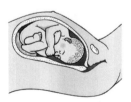 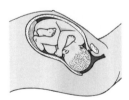

FIGURE 72

QUESTION 73

A primigravid 21-year-old woman at 39 weeks' gestation presents to the hospital complaining of labor. Membranes are intact. The cervix is dilated to 2 cm, 90% effaced and the vertex at 0 station. Contractions occur every 5–15 minutes and last about 15–25 seconds each. Two hours later, both her cervical exam and her contraction pattern remain unchanged. The fetal heart tracing is reassuring. The most appropriate next step is:

A. Cesarean section

B. Augmentation of labor with oxytocin

C. Radiographic pelvrimetry

D. Reexamine in 1 hour

E. Amniotomy and placement of internal monitors

QUESTION 74

A 19-year-old primigravid at 40 weeks' gestation has been in labor for the last 8 hours. Fetal heart tones have a baseline of 135/min with normal variability, multiple accelerations and no decelerations. She has been completely dilated for the last hour, and with pushing, has descended from a +1 station to a +3 station at present. The vertex is direct occiput anterior. Your next course of action is to recommend:

A. Forcep-assisted vaginal delivery

B. Vacuum-assisted vaginal delivery

C. Continue to push

D. Pitocin augmentation

E. Cesarean section

QUESTION 75

You are performing the admission history and physical on an otherwise healthy 17-year-old woman who presents to Labor & Delivery for induction at 41 weeks' gestation. Her past medical history is unremarkable, and in reviewing her prenatal records, you note that no abnormalities were found on her initial prenatal physical exam at 8 weeks' gestation. On your admission physical, you note subtle systolic ejection murmurs heard best over the aortic valve region, and you rate it a 1 on a scale of 6. This murmur is most likely due to:

A. Increased cardiac size

B. Increased stroke volume

C. Decreased peripheral resistance

D. Decreased cardiac valvular resistance

E. Increased hematocrit in pregnancy

QUESTION 76

During normal pregnancy, thyroid function is associated with an increase in:

A. Free triiodothyronine (T3)

B. Basal metabolic rate of 50%

C. Thyroid stimulating hormone (TSH) transfer to the fetus

D. Protein binding of thyroid hormones

E. Elevated T3 resin uptake

QUESTION 77

Which of the following maternal serum concentrations is increased during normal pregnancy?

A. Calcium

B. Albumin

C. Creatinine

D. Bicarbonate

E. Cholesterol

QUESTION 78

Which of the following sets of test results is most consistent with the euthyroid state in pregnant women? (Values are expressed as increased or decreased relative to those in nonpregnant patients; T4 = total thyroxine, FT4I = free thyroxine index, T3RU = triiodothyronine resin uptake.)

A. T4 increased, FT4I increased, T3RU increased

B. T4 increased, FT4I increased, T3RU normal

C. T4 increased, FT4I normal, T3RU decreased

D. T4 normal, FT4I increased, T3RU decreased

E. T4 normal, FT4I normal, T3RU normal

QUESTION 79

All of the following are appropriate indications for immunization during pregnancy EXCEPT:

A. Chronic bronchial asthma during an anticipated influenza epidemic

B. Known exposure to hepatitis B

C. Puncture wound of the foot

D. Known exposure to mumps

E. Known exposure to hepatitis A

QUESTION 80

A primigravid at term presents in labor. Her pregnancy is complicated by the fact that she has a twin gestation. The most common presentation of these twins at delivery is:

A. Transverse/breech

B. Breech/transverse

C. Vertex/vertex

D. Vertex/breech

E. Breech/vertex

QUESTION 81

You are asked to evaluate a newborn at 1 minute of life. The infant is blue, with slow, irregular respirations and a heart rate of 80. There is some flexion of the extremities, and the infant grimaces when you suction the nares. The 1-minute Apgar score of this infant is:

A. 2

B. 4

C. 6

D. 8

E. 10

QUESTION 82

A 19-year-old woman with regular menses and a 28-day cycle now presents with 8 weeks of amenorrhea. If her last menstrual period was April 17, using Naegele's rule, you would anticipate that her estimated date of confinement (EDC) is:

A. January 17

B. January 24

C. July 24

D. February 17

E. January 10

QUESTION 83

A 25-year-old multipara at 38 weeks presents in early labor. Leopold maneuvers note a soft, ballotable structure at the symphysis, small parts along the patient's left side, fetal back along the patient's right side, and a hard mobile object in the right upper quadrant. The most likely presentation is:

A. Vertex

B. Transverse

C. Breech

D. Compound

E. Face

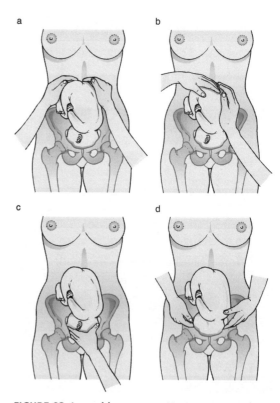

FIGURE 83 Leopold maneuver; Vertex presentation

QUESTION 84

During a routine urinalysis in pregnancy, which of the following is most likely to be a normal finding?

A. Glucosuria

B. Hematuria

C. Pyuria

D. Bacteriuria

E. Proteinuria

QUESTION 85

In a normal pregnancy at 16 weeks' gestation, which of the following has the highest alpha fetoprotein concentration?

A. Amniotic fluid

B. Fetal cerebrospinal fluid

C. Maternal serum

D. Fetal serum

E. Fetal urine

QUESTION 86

A 21-year-old nulligravid comes to your office for a routine physical exam. She is sexually active and has never had a Pap smear performed. She asks you what benefit the Pap smear has for her. You can tell her that having an annual Pap test screening is estimated to reduce a woman's chance of dying of cervical cancer by approximately:

A. 10%

B. 30%

C. 50%

D. 70%

E. 90%

QUESTION 87

In a complete hydatidiform mole, what are the origins of the chromosomes?

A. Maternal haploid

B. Paternal haploid

C. Maternal diploid

D. Paternal diploid

E. Maternal triploid

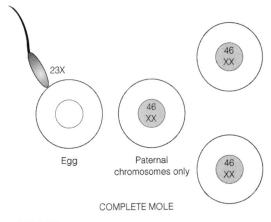

FIGURE 87

QUESTION 88

Which of the following pairs of HPV types is most commonly associated with the clinical picture seen in Figure 88?

A. 6/11

B. 16/18

C. 31/33

D. 39/45

E. 1/3

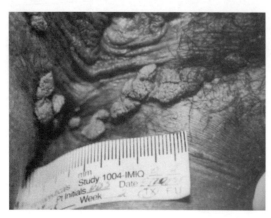

FIGURE 88

QUESTION 89

Due to an abnormal Pap smear suggestive of dysplasia, a woman is referred for evaluation. Your colposcopic exam is unsatisfactory since the entire transformation zone cannot be seen. The endocervical curettage result is negative for dysplasia, and the biopsy sample reveals CIN III. Your next step is to:

A. Repeat Pap smear.

B. Repeat endocervical curettage.

C. Repeat colposcopy and biopsy.

D. Perform conization of cervix.

E. Perform total abdominal hysterectomy.

QUESTION 90

On routine yearly exam of an otherwise healthy 45-year-old woman, you note a 1-cm erosive ulceration on the lower portion of the ecto-cervix. Which of the following is the most appropriate next step?

A. Punch biopsy of the lesion

B. Viral culture of the lesion for herpes simplex virus

C. Pap smear of the cervix

D. Dark field microscopy of a scraping of the lesion

E. Cold knife conization of the cervix

QUESTION 91

A 45-year-old woman is referred to your office for a Pap smear that is suspicious for malignancy. The cervix appears grossly normal on speculum exam. The next most appropriate procedure is:

A. Radical hysterectomy

B. Simple hysterectomy

C. Cervical cone biopsy

D. Cryotherapy of the cervix

E. Colposcopic directed biopsy

QUESTION 92

True statements concerning the diagnosis of an adnexal mass are the following, EXCEPT:

A. The diagnosis varies with the age of the patient.

B. In patients in the reproductive age period, a cystic mass larger than 5 cm should be explored immediately.

C. In premenarchal patients, most neoplasms are germ cell in origin and require surgical exploration.

D. In postmenopausal women, enlargement of the ovary is abnormal and should be considered malignant until proven otherwise.

E. In patients in the reproductive age period, a solid mass larger than 8 cm should be explored.

QUESTION 93

A 65-year-old woman comes to your office for a routine well-woman exam. Her last menstrual period was 15 years ago. She has not been on estrogen replacement therapy and now desires to start due to concerns about osteoporosis. On routine pelvic exam, you palpate a small uterus and cervix along with palpable ovaries bilaterally. Of the following, your next step in the management of this patient should be:

A. Start cyclic hormone replacement therapy: premarin 0.625 mg, 1–25 days; provera 10 mg, 16–25 days.

B. Start continuous hormone replacement therapy, premarin 0.625 mg and provera 2.5 mg qday.

C. Pelvic ultrasound

D. Dual photon densitometry for evaluation of bone density

E. Exploratory laparotomy

QUESTION 94

A postmenopausal woman comes to your office for advice because her best friend has been diagnosed with endometrial cancer. The patient is concerned that she too may develop the disease. You tell her that risk factors associated with endometrial cancer include the following, EXCEPT:

A. Nulliparity

B. Late menopause

C. DES exposure

D. Obesity

E. Polycystic ovarian disease

QUESTION 95

At the time of physical examination, detection of a lower-abdominal tumor in a 7-year-old girl is best accomplished by palpation of the abdomen coupled with:

A. Rectal examination

B. Vaginal examination

C. Rectovaginal examination

E. Abdominal auscultation and percussion

QUESTION 96

A 21-year-old patient comes to you for a pelvic examination and contraceptive counseling. She tells you she has never had intercourse and fears her vagina may be too small, even though she has used tampons for 3 years. You reassure her that her examination is normal. Which of the following approaches is the next step?

A. Gently dilate her hymen.

B. Demonstrate perineal sensory reflex.

C. Explain the normal physiology of the female sexual response.

D. Explain surgical procedures to enlarge the hymenal opening.

E. Prescribe dilators of progressive size.

QUESTION 97

During a routine office visit, a 19-year-old patient requests contraception. After discussing options, you prescribe an oral contraceptive. Several days later her father calls, asking if you prescribed oral contraceptives for his daughter. Your response is best guided by which of the following principles?

A. Honesty

B. Beneficence

C. Confidentiality

D. Informed consent

E. Justice

QUESTION 98

A patient complains that her otherwise healthy 66-year-old husband takes longer to achieve an erection than he did at age 40. You advise that:

A. At his age, sexual response is naturally slower.

B. He makes an appointment with a sex therapist.

C. He takes 20 mg of methyltestosterone daily.

D. She uses psychogenic stimulation.

E. He makes an appointment with a urologist.

QUESTION 99

A patient diagnosed as having a fetus with tri-somy 18 asks that you do not share this finding with her family. You may discuss her tests with:

A. Her husband

B. Her mother

C. Her father

D. No one

E. Her son

QUESTION 100

Which approach is most appropriate when examining the abdomen and genitals of a tick-lish child?

A. Divert the child's attention to a picture in the examining room.

B. Place the child's hands on top of yours for the duration of the examination.

C. Apply increased pressure to the abdomen until the ticklish sensation abates.

D. Ask the child's parent to hold the child still for the duration of the examination.

E. Ask your office assistant to hold the child still for the duration of the examination.

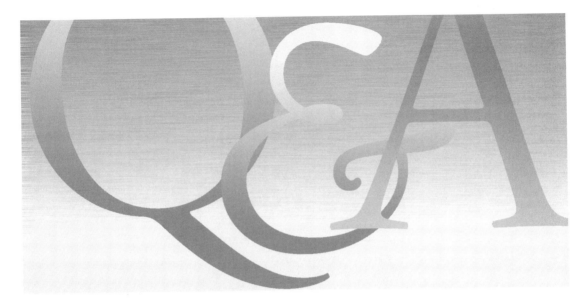

BLOCK **ONE**

ANSWERS

ANSWER 1

D. Given the prior cesarean section, the sudden onset of repetitive variable decelerations along with the sudden loss of fetal station is highly suspicious for uterine rupture. This occurs in about 0.5–1% of all women undergoing a trial of labor with a prior low transverse segment cesarean section. Classical uterine incisions have a much higher risk of uterine rupture, and labor is contraindicated in these women. Since uterine rupture can be catastrophic for both the mother and fetus, women who wish a trial of labor should deliver at a facility where emergency cesarean deliveries can be performed in a prompt and timely fashion.

A. Abruption is often associated with uterine pain and bleeding, but should not be accompanied by a loss of fetal station.

B. Previa is more often associated with painless vaginal bleeding. Also, the placenta would have been palpated during your pelvic exam.

C. Uterine hyperstimulation can be associated with late decelerations and uteroplacental insufficiency. No loss of fetal station should occur.

E. Cord prolapse would be palpable on pelvic exam. Loss of fetal station will increase this risk of this complication. Prolapse is not associated with bleeding and persistent pelvic pain.

ANSWER 2

E. The position of the fetal vertex is determined by the location of the fetal occiput relative to the maternal pelvis. When the sagittal suture is in the anterior-posterior axis of the pelvis, with the occiput closest to the symphysis, the vertex is considered to be occiput anterior (OA). When the sagittal suture is in the transverse axis of the pelvis, the vertex is either right or left occiput transverse (ROT, LOT). In this diagram, the occiput, as noted by the triangular shape of the posterior fontanelle, is to the patient's left side and posterior. The anterior fontanelle is anterior and to the patient's right. Since the landmark is the occiput, the position is left occiput posterior.

A. See Figure 2A.

B. See Figure 2B.

C. See Figure 2E.

D. See Figure 2C.

ANSWER 3

A. Due to the large overlap between a normal fetus and a fetus with trisomy 21 or 18, low alpha fetoprotein values should not be repeated, as the second value is more likely to be reported as normal (regression to the mean). Most patients now receive a triple screen, which includes AFP, HCG, and uE3. This triple screen test looks at the age-related risk for aneuploidy for each of the markers and then predicts a composite risk for both trisomy 21 and trisomy 18. With the triple screen, about 60–70% of all trisomy 21 pregnancies can be detected prenatally. In trisomy 18, all three values are low. Trisomy 13 cannot be screened by a low MSAFP.

B. Triploidy is not associated with a low MSAFP.

C. Twin pregnancy is often associated with an elevated MSAFP when compared to a singleton pregnancy.

D. Open neural tube defects are associated with an elevated MSAFP value.

E. Trisomy 13 cannot be routinely detected by the MSAFP value, unlike trisomies 18 and 21.

ANSWER 4

B. In an automobile accident, even with a restrained passenger, the gravid uterus in the third trimester will have a rapid deceleration within the abdominal cavity. This shear force can increase the risk of a placental abruption, as well as uterine rupture. Most cases of abruption occur within 24 hours of the accident. In this case, with absent fetal heart tones, a tense abdominal wall, and clinical evidence of hypovolemia, one should suspect the more serious condition of uterine rupture. With her vital sign changes, at least 1500–2000 cc or more of blood have been lost. Evaluation and correction of DIC as well as maternal blood volume replacement are indicated. Cesarean delivery of the fetus must be expedited since the blood loss will continue until the uterus is repaired.

A. Ruptured spleen can definitely be associated with significant hemorrhage and shock. Since the lower portion of her abdomen is tender, the diagnosis is more likely to be from a pelvic origin.

C. Perforated viscus is uncommon without penetrating trauma.

D. Abruption is a common occurrence in abdominal trauma of this nature. Due to the absent heart tones, tense abdomen, and signs of significant hypovolemia, uterine rupture is more likely.

E. Ruptured bladder should not be associated with absent fetal heart tones.

ANSWER 5

C. If a woman is nonimmune to rubella, then the risk of congenital rubella syndrome is 20% for a primary infection in the first trimester. Cataracts, patent ductus arteriosus, and deafness are the most common findings. In this case, she is coming to you within a few days of having an exanthem; if the patient's rubella IgG shows immunity, then the rash was not due to rubella. If she is rubella IgG negative, then obtain an IgM titer.

A. Rubella infection in an adult can be a mild viral exanthem. This finding should never be ignored in a pregnant female.

B. No diagnosis of the condition has been made at this time.

D. Streptococcal pharyngitis is usually associated with a fever, lymphadenopathy, and pharyngeal symptoms.

E. Toxoplasmosis is not associated with a maculopapular rash.

ANSWER 6

D. Diagnosis of intrauterine infection is usually based on maternal fever, maternal or fetal tachycardia, uterine tenderness, foul odor of the amniotic fluid, and leukocytosis. Bacteremia occurs in only 10% of cases. Once membranes are ruptured, the presence of a fever (100.4°F) in the absence of any other explanation for the elevated temperature should strongly suggest chorioamnionitis. Amniocentesis can assist in the diagnosis, when no other clinical signs are present besides a fever. The presence of bacteria in the amniotic fluid, or a fluid glucose level of less than 15 mg/dl, is presumptive evidence for infection. Interleukin 6 has the highest sensitivity of any diagnostic test.

A. Elevations in maternal leukocyte count can occur for a wide variety of reasons in pregnancy, including labor. It is not a reliable diagnostic finding.

B. Maternal tachycardia is a nonspecific finding and can also be associated with a wide variety of conditions.

C. Uterine tenderness is not always present and may be a late finding in the condition.

E. Maternal bacteremia occurs in only 10% of cases.

ANSWER 7

D. These are examples of repetitive late decelerations. Late decelerations are felt to be consistent with uteroplacental insufficiency. This can be due to a number of reasons, including the following: the maternal circulation is not adequately perfusing the placental bed; maternal hypoxia; inadequate exchange across the placental bed (abruption, infarct); and also inadequate fetal perfusion of the placenta. Since this is a recent change in the prior character of the fetal heart tracing and since the patient is on oxytocin infusion, allowing intrauterine resuscitation would be the most optimal choice. Should no improvement in the fetal condition occur, then the next step after this would be delivery.

A. Instrumented vaginal delivery is never indicated before the cervix is completely dilated.

B. Cesarean delivery would be indicated if measures to allow intrauterine resuscitation are unsuccessful (left lateral position, supplemental oxygen to the mother, discontinue contractions).

C. Amnioinfusion is appropriate for repetitive variable decelerations due to oligohydramnios. Its use for diluting thick meconium to decrease the incidence of meconium aspiration syndrome is controversial.

E. At present, repetitive late decelerations must be evaluated and measures undertaken to improve the fetal heart tracing. It is possible in the future, with the use of fetal pulse oximetry, that in some conditions this heart tracing can be further observed without intervention.

ANSWER 8

C. Although this patient has had a prior cesarean section, the possibility of a uterine scar separation is low. With the presence of ruptured membranes, a complete previa is unlikely. Although the uterus is tender, the patient is afebrile. There is literature to suggest that prolonged preterm ROM is associated with an increased risk of abruptio placentae.

A. Ruptured membranes with a complete previa is very unlikely.

B. Chorioamnionitis can be a complication of prolonged preterm rupture of membranes. It can be associated with contractions and uterine pain, but is usually not associated with vaginal bleeding.

D. Uterine scar separation can occur with a prior cesarean, but usually occurs in active labor. This patient is showing signs of early uterine activity at 32 weeks' gestation, making this diagnosis unlikely.

E. HELLP syndrome is hemolysis, elevated liver enzymes, and low platelets.

ANSWER 9

E. These are examples of early decelerations and are felt to be due to head compression. Increased intracranial pressure causes local changes in cerebral artery blood flow, leading to a reflexive bradycardia mediated by the vagal nerve. Although not all authors agree that this class of decelerations is distinct from variable decelerations, there is good evidence to suggest that early decelerations are not associated with fetal asphyxia. Early decelerations are most often seen around 4–6 cm of cervical dilation and should not have any associated tachycardia, loss of variability, or other heart rate changes.

A. Instrumented vaginal delivery is never indicated before the cervix is completely dilated.

B. Cesarean delivery would be indicated if evidence of uncorrectable fetal hypoxia should develop.

C. Amnioinfusion is appropriate for repetitive variable decelerations due to oligohydramnios. Its use for diluting thick meconium to decrease the incidence of meconium aspiration syndrome is controversial.

D. There is no evidence of uteroplacental insufficiency. Thus, no intervention is required.

ANSWER 10

C. The use of oral beta adrenergic tocolytics is controversial. In order to reach a therapeutic level, significant maternal side effects are usually seen, the most common of which are cardiovascular and metabolic. Resting tachycardia and a murmur of increased flow are usually present. The development of arrhythmias or pulmonary edema usually requires stopping therapy and switching to another class of tocolytic agent. Oral doses are given every 2–4 hours and continued until 34–36 weeks' gestation.

A. In order to reach a therapeutic dose of an oral tocolytic, cardiovascular side effects are commonly present as a result. If a patient has no contractions and no elevation in pulse, then the oral tocolytic probably is not required.

B. See the answer to A.

D. See the answer to A. The patient does not have an arrhythmia.

E. See the answer to A. Intervals longer than every 4 hours are usually not effective with oral terbutaline as a tocolytic.

ANSWER 11

C. Paternal diabetes has a genetic risk to the child, but does not pose any risk during pregnancy and delivery compared to other normal infants. If a patient is a gestational diabetic with a macrosomic fetus and a prior shoulder dystocia, a cesarean delivery is indicated.

A. This is probably the greatest risk for another shoulder dystocia. If her prior delivery resulted in a dystocia (especially if the child has permanent sequelae), then most obstetricians would proceed with an elective cesarean delivery.

B. Maternal obesity is associated with larger birth weights and an increased risk of complicated delivery.

D. Prolonged second stage can be a warning feature of an impending shoulder dystocia.

E. Fetal macrosomia increases the risk of complicated vaginal delivery, especially when the fetal weight is over 4500 g.

ANSWER 12

E. Eisenmenger's syndrome is one where there is communication between the systemic and pulmonary system, along with increased pulmonary vascular resistance, either to systemic level or above systemic level (right to left shunt). A would-be mother must be informed that to become pregnant would incur a 50% risk of dying. Even if she survives, fetal mortality approaches 50% as well.

A. Severe symptomatic aortic stenosis has a mortality in pregnancy of about 20%. Prevention of reduction in preload is necessary in all obstructive cardiac lesions. Balloon valvuloplasty can be done in pregnancy.

B. Due to the increased blood volume and cardiac output in pregnancy, mitral stenosis can lead to severe pulmonary edema. Balloon valvuloplasty can be done in pregnancy.

C. Ebstein anomaly is a malformation of the tricuspid valve. It is usually not associated with maternal mortality.

D. Atrial-septal defects rarely cause complications in pregnancy, labor, or delivery.

ANSWER 13

C. With the hypercoagulable state of pregnancy combined with her history of antiphospholipid antibody syndrome, this patient most likely has developed a venous thrombosis leading to a pulmonary embolus. Although the chest radiograph, electrocardiogram, and arterial blood gas are part of the routine workup of chest pain, the diagnosis is made by either a ventilation perfusion scan, spiral CT scan, or pulmonary angiography. Since the thrombus may be in the pelvis, doppler studies of the lower extremities may miss the source of emboli.

A. Often in a pulmonary embolus, the chest radiograph has no significant findings.

B. An electrocardiogram is not conclusive in diagnosing a pulmonary embolus. Signs of right ventricular strain may be present.

D. Emboli to the lung in pregnancy may be from a pelvic origin, so a lower extremity doppler may miss the source of the emboli.

E. An arterial blood gas will confirm arterial blood hypoxia, but this finding can occur in a wide variety of pulmonary and cardiac conditions; it is only suggestive for a pulmonary embolus.

ANSWER 14

A. Of all the non-Rh(D) red blood cell antigens, anti C, anti Kell, and to a lesser extent anti E are all capable of producing hemolytic disease as severe as that of anti D. Anti Lewis and Anti-P antibodies are IgM and do not cross the placenta (Kell antibodies include: k, K, Kp, Js). Note: A mnemonic that students often learn is Duffy dies, Kell, Kidd kill, Lewis lives.

B. Anti E is of intermediate danger for hemolytic disease. This antibody is usually of low titer.

C. Anti M rarely produces hemolytic disease.

D. Anti Lewis is an IgM and does not cross the placenta. Also, Lewis antigens are poorly expressed on the fetal and neonatal erythrocytes.

E. Anti P is an IgM and does not cross the placenta.

ANSWER 15

D. Late decelerations as a rule generally indicate uteroplacental insufficiency. A positive CST indicates that late decelerations are present on at least 50% of the contractions. This, along with the absence of variability, as well as other measures consistent with chronic growth restriction (oligohydramnios and weight <10th percentile), is an indication for immediate delivery. Since the Bishop score indicates an unripe cervix, this would be best done by performing a cesarean section.

A. Fetal karyotype is important for the workup of a symmetric IUGR fetus. This is the picture of uteroplacental insufficiency.

B. Fetal blood pH will not aid in the management of this patient. Immediate delivery is the answer.

C. A positive CST with an unripe cervix and IUGR at 38 weeks is managed by immediate delivery. Further fetal testing is not warranted.

E. This fetus needs delivery this day. Further delay may lead to stillbirth or other serious sequelae.

ANSWER 16

C.

A. This is seen in meningococcemia.

B. Allergic reactions do not appear 6 hours after administration of the medication.

D. Secondary bacteremia will not make the lesions painful. Chills, malaise, and fever can be seen with bacteremia.

E. Condyloma lata is one of the lesions of secondary syphilis, not human papilloma virus.

ANSWER 17

D. Division before day 4: diamniotic, dichorionic. Division during day 4–8: diamniotic, monochorionic. Division during day 8–12: monoamniotic, monochorionic. Division after day 12: conjoined. Acardiac twins only occur in monochorionic with delayed cardiac function in one twin, with arterial anastamosis leading to reversed arterial perfusion and absence of development of the heart tube. (TRAP: twin reversed arterial perfusion syndrome.)

A. Occurs before day 4.

B. Occurs between day 4 and 8.

C. This is where the cord inserts into the membrane away from the placental disc. It is more common in twin gestation than in singleton.

E. Acardiac twins are monochorionic twins, where the heart of one twin does not develop. This is a very rare condition.

ANSWER 18

B. Complete uterine inversion after delivery is typically due to excessive cord traction with a fundal placenta. Accreta and the use of magnesium may increase the risk of this complication. Life threatening hemorrhage and profound hypotension may rapidly occur. Prompt treatment is necessary to prevent a possible fatal outcome. Immediate replacement of the uterus should be attempted. While attempting this maneuver, large bore intravenous lines must be placed and adequate fluid resuscitation started. If successful, then uterotonic agents should be given. If unsuccessful, then various agents to relax the uterus may be necessary.

A. Intraabdominal hemorrhage will not be visible from the vagina.

C. Retroperitoneal hemorrhage will not be visible from the vagina.

D. The uterus will be soft and boggy, not firm as in this case.

E. Uterine rupture can have significant bleeding, but a mass will not be seen.

ANSWER 19

E. The internal iliac branches into an anterior and a posterior division. The posterior division gives rise to the superior gluteal, iliolumbar, and lateral sacral. The anterior division gives off the obturator, internal pudendal, uterine, superior and inferior vesicle, vaginal branches, and the obliterated umbilical artery. The middle and inferior rectal arteries arise off of the internal pudendal. The superior rectal is the final branch of the inferior mesenteric. The external pudendal arises off of the external iliac at the level of the inguinal ligament (along with the deep inferior epigastric and circumflex iliac, and sometimes the aberrant obturator).

A. See above explanation.
B. See above explanation.
C. See above explanation.
D. See above explanation.

ANSWER 20

D. Tanner stage 1 is defined as the prepubertal breast. The presence of a breast bud becomes stage 2. As the breasts develop and become conical, they are Tanner stage 3. When the areola elevates off of the breast mound, then stage 4 is reached. Tanner stage 5 is the mature adult breast contour.

A. See above answer.
B. See above answer.
C. See above answer.
E. See above answer.

ANSWER 21

B. The blood returning to the fetus from the placenta has the highest oxygen concentration. Blood in the umbilical vein travels through the ductus venosus into the inferior vena cava and into the right atrium. Most of this flow tends to go through foramen ovale into the left atrium and eventually out the ascending aorta. Blood returning from the heart via the superior vena cava tends to go through the tricuspid valve and out the pulmonary trunk, then through the ductus arteriosus into the aorta. Thus, higher oxygenated blood is found in the proximal aorta, which is supplying the head and neck.

A. Abdominal aorta is a mixture of blood from the placenta and blood returning from the body, since this artery is postductal.

C. This artery is taking blood to the placenta from the fetus.

D. The pulmonary artery is taking blood from the right ventricle. Due to the direction of flow, most of this blood is coming from the superior vena cava and is less oxygenated than the aortic arch.

E. This will have the same oxygen level as the abdominal aorta and the umbilical artery.

ANSWER 22

E. The arcuate line is the lower border of the transversus abdominus muscle. Below this line, the rectus abdominus is adjacent to the peritoneum; above it, the transversus is adjacent to the peritoneum.

A. Pyramidalis is external to and at the lower border of the rectus abdominus muscle.

B. Below the arcuate line, the rectus muscle is adjacent to the peritoneum.

C. External oblique is external to the internal oblique.

D. Internal oblique is external to the transversus abdominus.

ANSWER 23

B. Human chorionic gonadotropin doubles every 1.2–2 days in early pregnancy, with its peak being reached at 7–9 weeks after fertilization. It then declines to a plateau level for the remainder of the gestation.

A. See explanation.

C. See explanation.

D. See explanation.

E. See explanation.

ANSWER 24

B. Organogenesis is the most susceptible time during pregnancy for the fetus. Gestational age of maximal embryonic susceptibility to teratogens, week 6.

A. See explanation.

C. See explanation.

D. See explanation.

E. See explanation.

ANSWER 25

C. Overall, trisomy as a group accounts for 50% of all first trimester abortuses (of which trisomy 16 is the most common). Mono-somy X is the most frequent single anomaly found. Diploid of androgenetic origin is associated with gestational trophoblastic neoplasias such as complete and partial molar pregnancy.

A. An uncommon finding in abortuses.

B. An uncommon finding in abortuses.

D. Haploid of paternal origin will be a 23X or a 23Y.

E. Diploid of paternal origin is associated with complete molar pregnancy.

ANSWER 26

D. The most common cause of secondary amenorrhea is anovulation. Since she had a vaginal delivery 2 years ago, she has not had a prolonged exposure to unopposed estrogen, so the likelihood of an endometrial malignancy is very low. The most common finding is proliferative endometrium in this case. An Arias Stella reaction is found in pregnancy; it is the hypersecretory gland appearance seen on histopathology.

A. There have been only 2 years since her last delivery. It is unlikely that she has developed an estrogen induced neoplasia in that time frame.

B. See answer to A.

C. See answer to A.

E. This is the hypersecretory reaction to pregnancy.

ANSWER 27

A. This patient is demonstrating signs of increased androgen production. As her secondary sexual characteristics started appearing at age 6, she has, by definition, had a heterosexual precocious puberty. Since a cervix is present, the Mullerian system must have developed, meaning that the gonad is not testes, and that there is no Y component to her sex chromosomes. Her most likely sex chromosome pattern is XX.

B. The presence of a Y chromosome would lead the gonad to develop into testes. Anti-Mullerian hormone would be produced, and no cervix/uterus/fallopian tubes would develop.

C. See answer to B.

D. See answer to B.

E. See answer to B.

ANSWER 28

D. Complete androgen insensitivity syndrome is due to a congenital lack of androgen receptors. The patient never develops the Mullerian system since the gonad produces anti-Mullerian hormone (AMH or MIF) from the Sertoli cells during organogenesis. Although the patient has a male level of testosterone and male levels of estrogen, since the androgens are not recognized, the breasts develop due to the presence of estrogens. Without androgens, these patients often have sparse to no sexual hair. As the gonad is an XY gonad, it must be removed to prevent the risk of malignant transformation; this is rare prior to puberty, so it can be removed after normal pubertal development has occurred (most common malignancy is a gonadoblastoma).

A. One would see the effects of excess androgen: hair growth, virilization, etc.

B. The vagina would be behind the imperforate hymen and not visible. If menses has begun, then there would be a bluish bulging mass (vagina full of old menstrual blood).

C. A uterus is present in Turner syndrome.

E. Although a uterus is absent in this syndrome, sexual hair should be present since there is no defect in either androgen production or in androgen receptors.

ANSWER 29

E. After pregnancy, anovulation is the most common cause of secondary amenorrhea in a reproductive age woman. Asherman's syndrome is usually associated with a prior uterine curettage.

A. This is a rare cause of amenorrhea.

B. This is often secondary to intrauterine trauma (dilation and curettage, infection, etc.).

C. Although this can be a cause, it is uncommon.

D. Prolactinomas are rare causes of amenorrhea. They are often associated with galactorrhea.

ANSWER 30

D. The number one reason for absence of periods in a sexually active woman is pregnancy. Although this is not yet by definition secondary amenorrhea (>6 months of amenorrhea in a woman who has had prior menses), ruling out pregnancy is the first step that should be taken.

A. This would be ordered in a patient with galactorrhea and oligomenorrhea or amenorrhea.

B. This is not a usual test in the workup of amenorrhea.

C. Although abnormalities in thyroid function can lead to amenorrhea, in a patient with normal cycles until 3 months ago, this diagnosis would be unlikely.

E. This patient has no other symptoms of premature menopause (hot flashes etc.).

ANSWER 31

B. This is a young woman with normal height and normal breast and sexual hair development. The lack of a menstrual period is due either to a lack of the uterus or a blockage in the outlet of the menstrual efflux. The large suburethral bluish bulge, which can be palpated rectally as a midline mass, is a vagina full of menstrual blood (hematocolpos). The treatment is to incise the imperforate hymen and allow for normal menstrual flow. These young women are at higher risk for endometriosis. A transverse vaginal septum is higher in the vagina and is due to a failure of canalization of the sinovaginal bulb in utero.

A. A transverse vaginal septum is due to failure of the sinovaginal bulb to canalize during embryogenesis. This would be farther back in the vaginal vault.

C. No secondary sexual characteristics should be present.

D. Absence of androgen receptors would mean that there should not be any sexual hair.

E. This will lead to ambiguous genitalia at birth and heterosexual precocious puberty.

ANSWER 32

D. 21-OH deficiency accounts for 95% of the cases of congenital adrenal hyperplasia. It is also the most frequent endocrine cause of neonatal death. With severe forms, salt wasting, shock, and significant virilization occur. The genes for this enzyme are within the HLA complex on the short arm of chromosome 6.

A. This is one of the causes of congenital adrenal hyperplasia, but it is much less common than 21 alpha hydroxylase deficiency.

B. This enzyme converts pregnenolone to progesterone as well as 17 OH pregnenolone to 17 OH progesterone, as well as DHEA to androstenedione.

C. This converts androstenedione to testosterone and estrone to estradiol.

E. This converts 17 OH pregnenolone to DHEA and 17 OH progesterone to androstenedione.

ANSWER 33

E. In pregnancy, progesterone is produced by the corpus luteum followed by the placenta. Exogenous progesterone will not lead to withdrawal bleeding. In ovarian failure as well as pituitary failure, no estrogen stimulation of the endometrium exists, and progesterone cannot cause withdrawal bleeding. With Mullerian agenesis, there is no endometrium. Polycystic ovarian syndrome has an abundance of circulating estrogen, so the endometrium will proliferate.

A. Progesterone withdrawal will not occur since the corpus luteum is producing progesterone. The placenta will take over, starting at 7 weeks, and will be the sole producer of progesterone by 12 weeks.

B. No estrogen will be produced; no proliferation of the endometrium will occur.

C. Without gonadotropin stimulation, there will not be enough estrogen to stimulate the endometrial lining.

D. There is no uterus, thus no bleeding.

ANSWER 34

D. The luteal phase of the menstrual cycle is about 14 days in most women. Differences in cycle length are due to differences in the proliferative phase length. The reason that the cervical mucus is progestational is that the test was done 6 days too early. (A postcoital test is done at ovulation, which occurs 14 days prior to the NEXT menstrual period.) The correct thing to do is to repeat the test 6 or 7 days earlier on the next cycle.

A. Since the test was done at the wrong time of the cycle, no assessment of male factor can be made at this time.

B. See answer to A.

C. Although estrogen may change the nature of the cervical mucus, the test was done at the wrong time in the cycle.

E. The basal body temperature chart indicates ovulation (biphasic); so there is no benefit at this time for clomiphene citrate therapy.

ANSWER 35

C. This is the classic picture of "polycystic ovarian disease." The name of course is a misnomer, since the ovarian findings are simply a manifestation of the disease process and not the cause. On exam, she clearly has an abundance of estrogenic mucus, so a serum estradiol level would not be helpful. Hirsutism, acanthosis nigricans, hyperandrogenism, and insulin resistance are classic features of this syndrome.

A. A ratio of less than 4.5 is consistent with insulin resistance.

B. Testosterone levels should be measured in the workup of hyperandrogenic states. It is possible that an ovarian or adrenal tumor could be the source of elevated androgens.

D. With a long history of unopposed estrogen, the endometrium is at risk for neoplasia.

E. Clomiphene citrate lowers the negative feedback of estrogen at the hypothalamus. This leads to an increase in the levels of FSH and LH. It is not effective in the hypoestrogenic patient.

ANSWER 36

D. With extensive tubal disease on both the HSG and laparoscopy, operative assistance will be needed in order for an egg to reach the uterine cavity. Due to the tubal disease, GIFT is not possible. ICSI is the treatment of choice for azoospermia and severe oligospermia. The patient is ovulatory based on her basal body temperature chart, so ovulation induction alone is not necessary. IVF with transcervical transfer of the embryo is the optimal treatment for this couple. With blastocyst transfer, the current success rates are above 50%.

A. The two tests of tubal function both demonstrate that it is highly unlikely for the egg to successfully transport down the tube. Thus, IUI will be of no benefit, since the sperm and egg will not meet.

B. ICSI is used for oligospermic and even some azospermic males to achieve fertilization.

C. Again, ovulation induction alone will not be successful if the tubes are blocked bilaterally.

E. This technique can only be used if there is tubal patency. The egg and sperm mixture is placed in the distal fallopian tube via laparoscopy. The tubes here are blocked.

ANSWER 37

B. Beginning in the midluteal phase, progesterone is secreted in a pulsatile fashion, occurring immediately following an LH pulse. Prior to ovulation, progesterone levels are less than 1 ng/ml, but reach a midluteal level of 10–20 ng/ml.

A. See explanation above. FSH stimulates the production of estrogen as well as the production of FSH receptors.

C. See explanation above. When peak levels of estradiol are achieved, the onset of the LH surge then occurs.

D. See explanation above. FSH stimulates secretion of inhibin from granulosa cells and, in turn, is suppressed by inhibin.

E. See explanation above. Activin is related to inhibin, but has an opposite effect (stimulates FSH release and GnRH receptor number).

ANSWER 38

C. Postmenopausal estrogen therapy has been shown to do all of the following except decrease the risk of ovarian cancer. Although 5 years use of oral contraceptives has been shown to reduce the risk of ovarian cancer, no such association has been shown with hormone replacement.

A. ERT clearly decreases the rate of bone loss in the postmenopausal woman.

B. In women without preexisting coronary heart disease, there is a decreased rate of coronary death in women taking ERT. Some recent data suggest, however, that women with preexisting heart disease may be at greater risk for the first few years of therapy.

D. Studies have shown that the rate of bowel cancer is less in women on ERT.

E. The tissues of the pelvic floor and perineum are sensitive to estrogen. With the drop in circulating estrogens due to menopause, atrophy will occur.

ANSWER 39

D. The normal stages of pubertal development in order are: thelarche (breast budding), pubarche (sexual hair), peak height growth velocity, and menarche. The age of pubertal change in the United States has been getting earlier, with breast development starting between the ages of 10 and 11 and menarche between the ages of 12 and 13. The mean interval from thelarche to menarche is 2.3 years, with a standard deviation of 1 year. If no secondary sexual characteristics occur by age 14, or no menarche by age 16.5, then the diagnostic workup of primary amenorrhea is necessary.

A. Thelarche is before pubarche.

B. Menarche is the final event in the process.

C. Peak height growth velocity is about 1 year before the onset of menarche.

E. Often the first bleeding is not ovulatory.

ANSWER 40

E. This picture is a classic example of a phenotypic Turner syndrome female. Ninety-nine percent of all monosomy X fetuses will spontaneously abort. Congenital lymphedema in utero leads to the development of a cystic hygroma along with many of the other visible external manifestations. About 60% of Turner patients have total loss of one X chromosome, the remainder have either a structural abnormality in one of the X chromosomes or mosaicism with an abnormal X. Other phenotypic findings include a high arched palate, renal abnormalities (horseshoe kidney, partial or complete duplication, etc.), and a low posterior hairline. One-third of these women will have cardiovascular abnormalities (coarctation of the aorta, bicuspid aortic valve, etc.). Autoimmune disorders such as Hashimoto's thyroiditis and Addison's disease are common. The general recommendations are that gonadotropin levels are the first test indicated when the clinical picture of a classic Turner syndrome patient presents. A karyotype will confirm the diagnosis and help determine further recommendations should any Y chromosomal elements exist.

A. This patient will require hormone replacement therapy as she has no ovaries. It is not, however, the next step in the evaluation.

B. Growth hormone therapy in childhood has been suggested to allow these patients to approach near normal height in adulthood. It is controversial at present.

C. As no secondary sexual characteristics due to estrogen have appeared, an estradiol level will not be required.

D. Pelvic ultrasound may demonstrate tissue in the region of the adnexa. The streak gonads measure about 0.5 by 2.0 cm.

ANSWER 41

D. Leiomyomas are generally found only in the reproductive age group. Since they tend to regress after menopause and often grow during pregnancy, estrogen is felt to be stimulatory to their growth. GnRH analogs can be used to create a pseudomenopausal state and suppress their growth.

A. Leiomyomas are much more common in women of African-American descent.

B. Ultrasound is the most common diagnostic test done. The classic whorl-shaped lesions can be easily seen by this modality along with their location in the uterus.

C. Most women with fibroids are not infertile, but there is an association with fibroids and infertility.

E. Most women with fibroids do not have any problems with menorrhagia, pain, infertility, or other conditions.

ANSWER 42

D. The main mechanism of the contraceptive action of copper bearing IUDs in the human is as a spermicide. This effect is caused by a local, sterile, inflammatory reaction produced by a foreign body. There is a thousand-fold increase in the number of leukocytes in the washings of the endometrial cavity after the IUD is placed. This causes phagocytosis of sperm, and the tissue breakdown products of these leukocytes are toxic to both sperm and the blastocyst. Copper markedly increases this inflammatory reaction. Because of the spermicidal action of the copper IUD, few, if any, sperm reach the oviduct, and the ovum usually does not become fertilized.

A. Although there is a local inflammatory reaction, the main effect is spermicidal.

B. No effect on ovulation occurs from the copper IUD since it is nonhormonal.

C. See the answer to A.

E. No change in serum copper level occurs.

ANSWER 43

A. All of the contraceptive techniques decrease the risk of pregnancy in general. Since the overall rate of pregnancy is decreased, the rate of ectopic pregnancy is decreased as well. An intrauterine device decreases the chance of ectopic since its action is spermicidal (relative risk of 0.1 compared to no contraception). If a woman does become pregnant while using an IUD, however, she has a 7% chance that it is an ectopic.

B. See answer to A.

C. See answer to A.

D. See answer to A.

E. See answer to A. Since the IUD works mainly by a spermicidal action, it also decreases the risk of pregnancy in general. If a woman does become pregnant with the IUD, she has a 7% chance that she has an ectopic.

ANSWER 44

B. Currently, postcoital birth control can be done either with an IUD or with hormonal therapy. With OCPs, you need to give two doses, each of at least 100 μg of ethinyl estradiol (2 Ovral). Less than 2% of women will become pregnant with this dose (prevents 75% of expected pregnancies), and it can be given up to 72 hours after coitus. DES has a slightly higher success rate, but due to the significant side effect rate, compliance with this regimen is much less, making it less effective. An IUD is an option if there is no risk for sexually transmitted diseases, so it is not indicated after a sexual assault. Some countries also use two doses of 0.75 mg levonorgestrel, which has a similar success rate to the Ovral regimen. Note that the clinical pregnancy rate of unprotected midcycle coitus is about 7%.

A. IUDs can be used for emergency postcoital contraception, but are not indicated when the risk for a sexually transmitted disease is present.

C. A minimum of 100 μg of ethinyl estradiol in two divided doses needs to be given.

D. Significant side effects (nausea) make compliance with this regimen much less, making it less effective.

E. At this point, the fertilized ovum is still within the fallopian tube.

ANSWER 45

C. In a young woman, the most likely cause of this condition is fibrocystic changes in the breast. These are due to an exaggeration of the normal physiologic response of breast tissue to circulating ovarian hormones. Classic symptoms include cyclic bilateral breast pain, excessive nodularity, rapid change, and fluctuation in the size of cystic areas, increased tenderness, and occasionally nipple discharge. Symptoms are more common during the premenstrual phase of the cycle. Needle aspiration of the cyst is the first step. If a dominant mass remains after aspiration, tissue biopsy is mandatory.

A. If the mass does not resolve with aspiration, or recurs, then a mammography is indicated.

B. A solid or dominant mass needs tissue biopsy.

D. Although the cyst may decrease after menses, a symptomatic mass must be evaluated.

E. If a diagnosis of cancer has been made, this therapy may be appropriate.

ANSWER 46

D. All of these conditions are associated with dyspareunia. Inadequate vaginal lubrication, however, is the most common cause of pain with intercourse and can be due to a wide variety of causes.

A. Although a cause, it is not the most common. Psychosexual therapy may be of benefit to this patient.

B. When the uterosacral ligaments and cul-de-sac are involved, or due to pelvic adhesive disease, then intercourse can become painful. It is not the most common cause.

C. Has been associated with dyspareunia. Not a common cause.

E. See answer to B.

ANSWER 47

E. The cervical cap, more popular in Europe than in the United States, has a similar failure rate to the diaphragm (2 year pregnancy rate of 15–20%). It is much more effective in nulliparous than in parous women. About two-thirds of the failures are user related. It should only be used on women with normal Pap smears and should not be left in place more than 48 hours because of the possibility of ulceration, unpleasant odor, and infection.

A. See explanation.

B. See explanation.

C. See explanation.

D. See explanation.

ANSWER 48

C. Any smoker over the age of 35 has a significantly increased risk of myocardial infarction, stroke, and death if they are on oral contraceptive pills. Since she has heavy and painful menses, she is not an ideal candidate for the IUD. Endometrial ablation may lessen her menorrhagia, but it is not an accepted form of contraception. Norplant has no estrogen component; so it will not increase her risk of thromboembolic phenomena.

A. Due to her heavy, painful menses, not a good candidate for the IUD.

B. Smokers over 35 have an increased risk of MI and death when using estrogen-containing oral contraceptives.

D. This is not an accepted method of contraception. It may reduce her degree of menorrhagia.

E. Although this will successfully prevent pregnancy, contraception alone is not an acceptable indication for hysterectomy.

ANSWER 49

C. Routine health care screening is still necessary in this patient. This will include a yearly Pap smear, q5 year routine cholesterol screening, baseline mammography, and routine vital signs. Endometrial sampling is not required.

A. Routine initial mammography screening is indicated at age 40.

B. Yearly Pap tests are indicated. Should the woman be low risk and have three consecutive normal yearly Pap smears, then increasing the interval length up to q3 years may be appropriate.

D. Every 5 years cholesterol screening is indicated.

E. Routine vital signs are part of the necessary yearly health care screening.

ANSWER 50

D. The most likely diagnosis is a prolapsed sub-mucous fibroid. If this patient were 80 years old, presenting in the same fashion, one would be suspicious of a stromal sarcoma. Although this could be a carcinoma, the simplest and safest way to stop the bleeding is to remove the mass vaginally (ligate the stalk and then excise). The mass can be sent for pathologic evaluation with further therapy as indicated.

A. Although this would stop her bleeding, it carries a much higher risk to the patient (blood loss, ureteral injury, bladder injury). Should the mass turn out to be a malignancy, then the wrong procedure may have been done.

B. See answer to A.

C. Biopsy of the mass alone will not solve the bleeding. Since the stalk is visible and only 1.5 cm in diameter, then excision of the mass would be the best therapy.

E. High dose birth control pills can be used for dysfunctional uterine bleeding. Here, the bleeding is due to a prolapsed fibroid. OCPs will not affect her bleeding and pain.

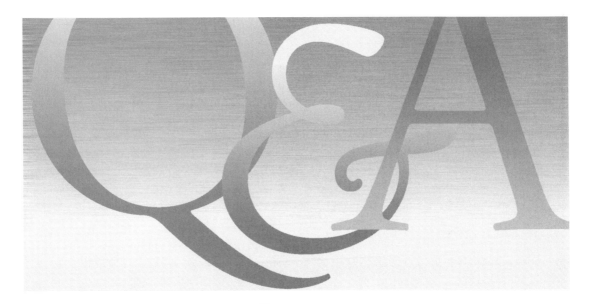

BLOCK TWO

ANSWERS

ANSWER 51

D. Dysmenorrhea is defined as a severe painful cramping sensation in the lower abdomen, often accompanied by other biologic symptoms, including sweating, tachycardia, headaches, nausea, vomiting, and diarrhea. All of these occur during or just before menses. The term primary dysmenorrhea is reserved for women with no obvious pathologic condition, and this is due to the effects of endogenous prostaglandins.

A. Dysmenorrhea in a 13-year-old is usually due to the effects of endogenous prostaglandins.

B. Usually, no visible peritoneal pathology can be found in primary dysmenorrhea.

C. Although OCPs have been used for this condition, they are not as effective as prostaglandin synthetase inhibitors.

E. This pain is debilitating to the patient. Reassurance with follow-up evaluation most likely will not decrease her pain and discomfort.

ANSWER 52

D. The most likely site of an ectopic is the ampulla. Cervical, ovarian, and abdominal ectopics are very rare. Cornual ectopics often present later, and the rupture can be much more catastrophic due to the vascularity of this portion of the uterus.

A. Cervical pregnancies can lead to massive bleeding. The cervix will often feel very large and can be tender. Methotrexate therapy may decrease the need for hysterectomy.

B. Cornual pregnancies often present later in gestation. When these rupture, due to their size and location near branches of the uterine arteries, the blood loss can be acute and massive.

C. Less common than ampullar ectopics.

E. See answer to C.

ANSWER 53

B. With her prior history of PID, her chances of tubal damage are significantly elevated. Since she is pregnant with an HCG titer over 2000 mIU/ml, an intrauterine gestation sac should have been seen on the endovaginal ultrasound. With the moderate amount of free fluid in the cul-de-sac, along with the pelvic pain and normal white count and temperature, the index of suspicion for an ectopic must be high.

A. The white count is normal and her temperature is normal as well. With a positive HCG titer, an ectopic should be the first suspicion.

C. This can cause free fluid in the cul-de-sac as well as pelvic pain. With her history of PID in the past, the presence of tubal damage is high; so one should be much more suspicious of an ectopic. At an HCG titer of 5,400, an IUP should have been seen.

D. Although a source of pelvic pain, with the HCG titer, absence of an IUP on ultrasound, and free fluid in the cul-de-sac, ectopic pregnancy should be the primary diagnosis.

E. Can be a source of pelvic pain. See answer to D.

ANSWER 54

D. The first day of the cycle is the first day of the menses. The length of the cycle is from the first day of one menses to the first day of the next menses. Many patients think that the length of the cycle is from the end of the menses to the beginning of the next. Thus, a number of women think that they have 21- to 23-day cycles.

A. Many patients count the days between periods as their cycle length. This will falsely shorten the length of their true cycle.

B. Even if the answer to this question is yes, there is no way to ascertain the actual length of their cycle.

C. See answer to A.

E. The last few days of a menses can be variable in length and degree of bleeding/spotting. It is less accurate to count this way than to count from the beginning of one cycle to the beginning of the next.

ANSWER 55

A. Bacterial vaginosis is due to an overgrowth of anaerobic bacteria, replacing the normal peroxide-producing lactobacillus species. The discharge is described as thin and gray-white in color. It is mildly adherent to the vaginal walls on speculum exam. In the presence of basic environment (semen, KOH), the aromatic amines are released, giving rise to the characteristic fishy odor.

B. In order to create an odor with a strong base, there must be aromatic amines present. These are created by certain anaerobic bacteria.

C. See answer to B.

D. See answer to B.

E. See answer to B.

ANSWER 56

C. The CDC recommendations for the treatment of PID with intravenous medications include (A) cefoxitin and doxycycline, (B) clindamycin and gentamicin. In treating an abscess, it is necessary to have anaerobic coverage by agents such as clindamycin or metronidazole. Quinolones with clindamycin can also be used. Aminoglycosides do not cover against anaerobes since their transport into the bacterial cell is coupled with oxidative phosphorylation.

A. With this regimen, Gram-negative coverage may not be appropriate.

B. With this regimen, anaerobic coverage may not be appropriate.

D. With this regimen, anaerobic coverage may not be appropriate.

E. With this regimen, anaerobic coverage may not be appropriate.

ANSWER 57

E. Molluscum is caused by a pox virus and is spread by direct contact. It is mildly contagious. The classic lesion is a small nodule, or domed papule with an umbilicated center. These lesions range from 1–5 mm in diameter and have a caseous material filling them. Treatment is excision with a dermal curette followed by chemical treatment of the base with Monsel's or trichloroacetic acid.

A. Sebaceous cysts are not umbilicated and are below the dermis.

B. This is a flat fleshy lesion of secondary syphilis, usually found on mucous membranes.

C. This is a flat papular dermatologic lesion. It is not umbilicated.

D. This is an exfoliative papular dermatologic lesion. It is not umbilicated.

ANSWER 58

D. Pelvic inflammatory disease (PID) has a high association with gonorrhea and chlamydia. After several days of inflammation, the bacterial flora is often polymicrobial. Pain, cervical motion tenderness, leukorrhea from the cervical os, fever, and leukocytosis are all common signs found when a patient presents with PID.

A. This is one of the criteria that is often used in making the diagnosis of pelvic inflammatory disease.

B. See answer to A.

C. See answer to A.

E. See answer to A. This is due to the inflammation of the tubes and peritoneum; moving the cervix from side to side will result in significant pain from the stretching of the inflamed peritoneum.

ANSWER 59

C. The fleshy lesions described are known as condyloma lata. Along with her generalized rash (which does not spare the palms and soles), this patient has the classic picture of secondary syphilis. Single dose benzathine penicillin is the standard therapy for primary, secondary, and early latent (latent of less than 1 year duration). Triple dose therapy is necessary for late latent.

A. This therapy can be used for HPV lesions. This patient has secondary syphilis.

B. See answer to A.

D. This therapy is used for late latent syphilis. This patient has secondary syphilis and only needs a single dose of benzathine penicillin.

E. This therapy is used to decrease the duration of herpes simplex infection.

ANSWER 60

D. This is the classic picture for toxic shock syndrome. Although it is more commonly associated with tampon usage, it can occur after use of a contraceptive sponge, diaphragm, or cervical cap. It can also occur postoperatively in a patient with gauze packing. Cultures are usually negative, though *Staphylococcus aureus* is the most common pathogen. An exotoxin is the causative agent for the systemic effects. Correction of circulatory compromise is the most important initial therapy in treating this condition. If a source exists for the bacteria, it must be removed as well (i.e., tampon, etc.).

A. In most cases of toxic shock syndrome, the causative agent will not be found in the blood stream.

B. This is not the typical presentation of disseminated gonococcemia.

C. The causative agent for the systemic effects is an exotoxin produced by the bacteria.

E. Correction of circulatory compromise and removal of the bacterial source are the most important initial therapies.

ANSWER 61

A. A mucopurulent cervicitis, along with urinary symptoms, makes one highly suspicious for *Neisseria gonorrhoeae*. Although all of the above tests would be helpful in determining the diagnosis, the only test that can aid you immediately is a Gram stain. The Gram stain has a sensitivity of only 60%, but a specificity of 95%. The key finding is a Gram-negative intracellular diplococcus.

B. Often with a gonococcal cervicitis, the peripheral white blood cell count is normal.

C. Chamydial testing of the cervical smear is not an immediate test.

D. Cervical culture on Thayer Martin medium is confirmatory, but is not an immediate test.

E. The urinary symptoms most likely are due to a gonococcal urethritis as well as a cervicitis. Routine dipstick urinalysis will not identify the pathogen involved.

ANSWER 62

C. In any woman over the age of 35, with abnormal uterine bleeding, the diagnosis of an endometrial malignancy must be entertained. With a postmenopausal woman having an endometrial stripe over 4 mm, cancer needs to be ruled out and tissue should be obtained. The simplest test is to proceed with an endometrial biopsy.

A. This therapy would be indicated as therapy for adenocarcinoma of the endometrium or for atypical endometrial hyperplasia. A diagnostic sampling of the endometrium is the first necessary test.

B. Although this test would lead to a diagnosis, an endometrial biopsy can be done more easily in the office with minimal discomfort.

D. This modality is used for the reproductive age female with severe symptomatic uterine bleeding in the absence of endometrial pathology.

E. A diagnosis of the endometrium must be made before hormonal therapy can be started in this case.

ANSWER 63

C. Management of an asymptomatic 45-year-old with leiomyomata: reexamine in 6 months. Leiomyomas are a frequent finding in a reproductive age woman. If they are asymptomatic (absence of pain, menorrhagia, urinary symptoms, gastrointestinal symptoms), and if they are small and not rapidly changing in size, then they can be followed. Since her last exam 1 year ago was reportedly normal, reexamination in less than 1 year would be appropriate.

A. Indicated for symptomatic fibroid uterus in a woman who does not desire fertility.

B. Necessary only if the woman is having abnormal uterine bleeding.

D. See answer to B.

E. Can be used for symptomatic leiomyomas in a reproductive age woman, but no more than 6 months of continuous therapy. This woman is without symptoms.

ANSWER 64

B. The most common cause for a cystic enlargement of the ovary in a reproductive age woman is a functional cyst (follicular or corpus luteum). These are thin walled and usually resolve or rupture spontaneously. Any cystic mass 6 cm or less can be followed for two cycles. Some texts recommend using oral contraceptive pills to decrease the gonadotropin stimulation of the ovary during this time, but there is no literature that shows any improvement over simple observation.

A. If the mass persists, further evaluation and possible surgical intervention is indicated. Laparoscopic surgery is less invasive and just as successful as laparotomy.

C. As most cystic masses in the adnexa are functional cysts that resolve spontaneously, no other workup is indicated at this time.

D. See answer to C. If the mass persists, an ultrasound would be the next step in the workup.

E. See answer to A.

ANSWER 65

B. Ovarian torsion may account for up to 3% of gynecologic emergencies requiring operative intervention. This usually occurs in a reproductive age woman who has an 8–12 cm benign mass of the ovary. Dermoids are the tumors most associated when a torsion has occurred, but paratubal and paraovarian cysts have the highest relative risk for torsion due to their thin stalk. If it is a benign cystic mass, and the ovary is not necrotic, the treatment of choice is a cystectomy with preservation of the remaining ovarian tissue. Preoperative doppler flow can be helpful in determining the viability of the adnexa.

A. Although right lower quadrant pain is commonly due to appendicitis, it is the sudden onset of cramping pain along with the lack of a fever that suggests ovarian torsion as the most likely etiology.

C. Urine pregnancy test being negative rules out ectopic.

D. Rupture of an ovarian cyst can cause peritoneal findings. With the 8-cm tender mass, a torsion is more likely.

E. It is unlikely that a woman would have been asymptomatic with a tuboovarian abscess prior to its rupture.

ANSWER 66

A. In a young child, if the straddle injury is nonpenetrating and associated with a non-expanding small vulvar hematoma, then ice packs and conservative therapy are preferred. In the presence of vaginal bleeding, an examination under anesthesia is required. The depth of many lacerations is greater than initially suspected and can involve neighboring organs and structures. Although a fall is the usual cause of a straddle injury in a young child, sexual abuse must always be considered in the differential diagnosis.

B. Having anyone, including the patient's mother, attempt to restrain the girl while she is being examined will often result in an unsatisfactory exam as well as emotional trauma.

C. See answer to B.

D. With the presence of vaginal bleeding, penetrating trauma must be ruled out.

E. If peritoneal contents are seen spilling into the vagina during the exam under anesthesia, then a laparotomy may be necessary.

ANSWER 67

A. Based on the exam findings in this multiparous woman, one would suspect that an anatomic stress incontinence picture is the most likely. If she had a fistula, the leaking would occur even at rest. As she is otherwise healthy, the likelihood of a neurogenic bladder (seen in diabetes, neuromuscular disorders, spinal cord injury) is small.

B. Urge incontinence, usually due to detrussor dyssynergia, has a hypercontractile bladder. The patient will sense the urge to void and often will not make it to the bathroom in time, as the spontaneous bladder contraction will cause urine loss. Anticholinergics are often used in this condition.

C. This condition will lead to leaking at all times, even at rest, since the defect is above the urethral sphincter.

D. See answer to B.

E. A neurogenic bladder will have overdistension and incomplete filling. With increased abdominal pressure, leaking can occur. Conditions such as chronic diabetes and spinal cord injury can cause this. Since she is otherwise healthy, this is unlikely.

ANSWER 68

B. The high level of estrogen is inhibitory to the production of milk by the breast despite the extremely high level of prolactin. After delivery of the fetus and placenta, the level of estriol decreases until the inhibitory effect is removed, at which time significant milk production begins (2–3 days).

A. Insulin levels elevate in pregnancy. This hormone, however, does not suppress lactation.

C. Total T4 levels rise in pregnancy due to an increase in thyroid hormone binding globulin. Free T4 levels stay essentially unchanged.

D. HPL increases free fatty acids, allowing glucose and amino acids to be conserved for use by the fetus.

E. Inhibin is produced by the placenta. Levels rise during pregnancy, causing a suppression of maternal gonadotropins.

ANSWER 69

B. The risk that she is a carrier is 2/3. Her parents must both be carriers. Since she is healthy, she is either a carrier (2/4) or homozygous normal (1/4), giving a 2/(1+2) or 2/3 risk of being a carrier. The carrier risk of the father is 1/22 (normal population risk). The risk of two carriers having an affected offspring is 1/4. Thus, the final risk is 2/3 times 1/22 times 1/4, which equals 1/132.

A. See explanation above.

C. See explanation above.

D. See explanation above.

E. See explanation above.

ANSWER 70

A. The most common form of vulvovaginitis is *Candida*. Only 20% of the patients will have a cottage cheese type of discharge. A KOH preparation will show hyphae.

B. Bacterial vaginosis will show clue cells on a wet mount. These epithelial cells demonstrate the classic findings of a clue cell: they have a ground glass appearance with irregular borders due to the large number of bacteria coating their surface, and with the application of KOH to the wet mount there is a characteristic fishy amine odor. The discharge tends to be gray and clings to the vaginal wall.

C. This discharge is often frothy, and when severe the cervix will appear strawberry red.

D. Often with chlamydia the patient is asymptomatic.

E. HPV can be associated with increased desquamation of the vaginal walls and cytolysis, but usually this is not curd-like in nature. Most HPV infections are not associated with a vaginal discharge.

ANSWER 71

D. In a susceptible patient, even pregnant, the standard therapy is to give the hepatitis B immune globulin to cover the needle stick exposure, followed by the vaccination. This vaccination is not a live vaccine, so it is not contraindicated in pregnancy.

A. Hepatitis-specific immune globulin and vaccination are required.

B. Immune globulin to cover the immediate exposure is also needed.

C. Hepatitis vaccine is required as well.

E. The risk of infection is high and can be prevented by the recommended therapy. Observation is not the standard care.

ANSWER 72

B. Engagement of the fetal head is defined by the biparietal diameter entering the pelvic inlet. Although 0 station is often used to imply engagement, this is only an estimation, since one cannot reach the pelvic inlet on a normal pelvic exam. If the pelvis is long, or the head very small, then the vertex could be engaged at a minus station. Conversely, if the pelvis is short, or the head very big, then engagement may not occur until a plus station has been achieved.

A. This is the definition of zero station, often used to imply engagement.

C. The biparietal diameter is the measurement used to define engagement.

D. See answer to A.

E. At this point, the fetal vertex is almost crowning (+4 station) and has engaged long before.

ANSWER 73

D. This is a patient in the latent phase of the 1st stage of labor. For a primigravid, this can last up to 20 hours before it is considered prolonged. At this point in time, there is no need for any intervention, since everything is normal. Often, these patients are even sent home and told to return when more active labor occurs.

A. The patient is in the latent phase of labor and the fetal condition is fine. No indication for cesarean exists at this point in time.

B. The patient is in the latent phase of labor and the fetal condition is fine. No indication for augmentation exists at this point in time.

C. The patient is in the latent phase of labor and the fetal condition is fine. There is no concern about the adequacy of the maternal pelvis.

E. The patient is in the latent phase of labor and the fetal condition is fine. No indication for amniotomy nor intervention exists at this point in time.

ANSWER 74

C. This patient is progressing in normal fashion. She is allowed up to 2 hours in the second stage and even longer if the heart tones are reassuring. There is no need to intervene, and one would anticipate that the patient will be having a normal spontaneous vaginal delivery within the next hour.

A. The patient has made adequate descent in the last hour. She can push for at least another hour and maybe more if the fetal condition remains reassuring. No indication for instrumental vaginal delivery is present.

B. The patient has made adequate descent in the last hour. She can push for at least another hour and maybe more if the fetal condition remains reassuring. No indication for instrumental vaginal delivery is present.

D. The patient has made adequate descent in the last hour. She can push for at least another hour and maybe more if the fetal condition remains reassuring. Since progress has been made, there is no need to augment the labor with pitocin.

E. The patient has made adequate descent in the last hour. She can push for at least another hour and maybe more if the fetal condition remains reassuring. No indication for cesarean delivery is present.

ANSWER 75

B. Maternal blood volume is up 40–50% by the start of the third trimester. Maternal stroke volume and cardiac output are up by a similar fraction, leading to an increase in turbulent flow with ventricular emptying. This gives rise to a flow murmur at the aortic valve. The hematocrit in pregnancy should decrease since the red cell mass only goes up 30% (physiologic anemia of pregnancy).

A. Ejection murmurs are due to the increase in turbulent flow.

C. Although peripheral resistance decreases, reaching a nadir in the second trimester, the murmur is still due to turbulent flow secondary to the 50% increase in cardiac output.

D. See answer to A.

E. The hematocrit decreases in pregnancy due to a relative increase in plasma volume relative to red cell mass.

ANSWER 76

D. TSH does not cross the placenta in significant amounts, but T4 transfer in early gestation may have a protective role in the early neural development of the fetus. Thyroid-binding globulin levels are increased, leading to an increase in the amount of bound thyroid hormone. Free thyroid hormone stays in the normal range, and total thyroid hormone levels are elevated. The T3 resin uptake is inversely proportional to the hormone binding capacity, so it decreases in normal pregnancy.

A. Stays essentially unchanged.

B. Basal metabolic rate remains essentially unchanged.

C. TSH does not cross the placenta in significant amounts.

E. The T3 resin uptake decreases since the percent of thyroid hormone that is bound has increased.

ANSWER 77

E. Albumin will decrease due to dilutional effects. Bicarbonate decreases due to increased renal excretion to correct for the respiratory alkalosis (blowing off more CO_2). Due to the 50% rise in GFR, the serum creatinine falls. Due to the decline in serum albumin, the total serum calcium concentration falls. Plasma levels of lipids increase during the latter part of pregnancy, the most marked rises occurring with triglycerides, cholesterol, and free fatty acids.

A. Serum albumin falls, and the total calcium concentration falls as well.

B. Serum albumin levels fall due to dilutional effects.

C. Creatinine falls due to a 50% increase in glomerular filtration rate. This occurs as early as 12 weeks' gestation.

D. Bicarbonate decreases as the kidney excretes more to compensate for the drop in CO_2 levels (due to increase in minute ventilation; renal compensation for a respiratory alkalosis).

ANSWER 78

C. Thyroid-binding globulin levels are increased, leading to an increase in the amount of bound thyroid hormone. Free thyroid hormone stays in the normal range, and total thyroid hormone levels are elevated. The T3 resin uptake is inversely proportional to the hormone-binding capacity, so it decreases in normal pregnancy.

A. FT4I should be normal, T3RU should be decreased.

B. See answer to A.

D. T4 is increased, FT4I is normal.

E. T4 is increased, T3RU is decreased.

ANSWER 79

D. Remember that live virus vaccines such as measles, mumps, and rubella are contraindicated. Inactive virus vaccines such as influenza are given only to those with serious underlying diseases. Tetanus is a toxoid vaccination.

A. Influenza is a killed virus vaccine and is safe in pregnancy.

B. Hepatitis B is not a live virus vaccine and is safe in pregnancy.

C. Tetanus vaccination is a toxoid, not a virus.

E. Prevention of hepatitis A does not require a live virus vaccine.

ANSWER 80

C. The most common presentation of twins at delivery is vertex/vertex followed next by vertex/breech.

A. Least common presentation

B. Less common presentation

D. Second most common presentation

E. Third most common presentation

ANSWER 81

B. The Apgar score is a useful tool in determining the need for infant resuscitation at both 1 minute and 5 minutes. It is not, however, a good tool to determine long term outcome. The five categories that the Apgar score evaluates are: heart rate, respiratory effort, muscle tone, reflex irritability, and color. 0, 1, or 2 points are awarded for each category, for a maximum score of 10. This infant scores 1 for heart rate, 1 for respiratory effort, 1 for muscle tone, 1 for reflex, and 0 for color, for a total score of 4 at 1 minute.

A. An Apgar score of 2 would be a blue limp infant, with no response to stimuli and a heart rate of less than 100 with minimal breathing effort. (or the same with a heart rate over 100 and no breathing effort.)

C. Infants with this Apgar score may need some stimulation and resuscitation efforts.

D. Infants with this Apgar score are usually vigorous and require no significant resuscitation efforts.

E. This would be a vigorous infant, with pink extremities, vigorous tone, respiration, heart rate, and good reflex. Most infants only score a 9 at best at 5 minutes.

ANSWER 82

B. Naegele's rule is used to estimate when 40 completed weeks of pregnancy have occurred. Add 7 days and subtract 3 months from the LMP will result in the EDC. This rule requires the woman to have regular cycles of normal length.

A. For this date to be her EDC, her LMP would have been April 10

C. For this date to be her EDC, her LMP would have been October 17

D. For this date to be her EDC, her LMP would have been May 10

E. For this date to be her EDC, her LMP would have been April 3

ANSWER 83

C. Leopold's can be used to assess the fetal lie. The gold standard is ultrasound, though a vaginal exam can help confirm the findings on abdominal exam. Only 3–4% of pregnancies at term present as nonvertex. External cephalic version can help reduce the number of cesarean sections done for this indication.

A. The cephalic pole should be palpable at the symphysis and the podalic pole at one of the upper quadrants.

B. No palpable pole should be noted at the symphysis.

D. This can be difficult to determine via Leopold maneuvers and is often detected only by pelvic exam.

E. This is usually detected by pelvic exam.

ANSWER 84

A. Due to the increase in glomerular filtration rate by 50%, the transport maximum for glucose can be reached at a much lower serum concentration. Occasional spillage of glucose in the urine is a normal finding in pregnancy.

B. Routine urinalysis should not have the presence of blood.

C. Routine urinalysis should not show evidence of infection.

D. Routine urinalysis should not show evidence of infection.

E. True proteinuria is abnormal in pregnancy and may either represent preeclampsia or an underlying renal abnormality.

ANSWER 85

D. Produced primarily in the fetal liver, alpha fetoprotein is the major oncotic protein in the fetus. It reaches a peak value in fetal serum at 12–14 weeks, at a level of about 3 mg/ml. The peak value in fetal amniotic fluid is around 40 µm/ml and occurs at or just after that in fetal serum. The maternal serum reaches its peak of 200 ng/ml at the end of the second trimester and begins to gradually decrease after 30 weeks. Thus, the concentration of AFP in the fetal serum is 10,000-fold greater than that in maternal serum.

A. The concentration of AFP in the amniotic fluid is less than that in fetal blood.

B. The concentration of AFP in the cerebrospinal fluid is less than that in fetal blood.

C. The concentration of AFP in the maternal serum is 10,000-fold less than that in fetal blood.

E. The concentration of AFP in the fetal urine is less than that of fetal blood. In cases of severe fetal nephrotic syndrome, fetal urine will have a high AFP concentration, and the MSAFP will often be significantly elevated (sometimes well beyond that found with a neural tube defect).

ANSWER 86

E. The use of the routine Pap smear as a screening tool for cervical cancer has helped to significantly decrease the number of women dying from this disease over the last 50+ years. The most common cancer caused death in women is now lung followed by breast, colorectal, ovary, and pancreas. In the world, cervical cancer remains the leading gynecologic cancer killer of women.

ANSWER 87

D. Complete mole. paternal diploid, 95% XX, 5% XY. Incomplete mole: triploid, with two sets of paternal origin, 69 XXY, etc. A complete mole does not have a fetus. Due to the high levels of HCG, it can be associated with hyperthyroidism, theca lutein cysts, and hyperemesis gravidarum. It can also be associated with preeclampsia in the first trimester.

ANSWER 88

A. Over 60 types of HPV have been identified. Types 6/11 are associated with genital condylomata and the minor CIN groups. When HPV 6/11 are found with CIN, the regression rate is high. Types 16/18 have a high association with cervical carcinoma and advanced cervical dysplasia.

B. These are the HPV serotypes that are commonly associated with cervical neoplasia, with 16 having the greatest association with invasive squamous cell carcinoma.

C. These have also been associated with cervical neoplasia.

D. Not associated.

E. Not associated with genital lesions.

ANSWER 89

D. Conization of the cervix should be performed because the transformation zone or the lesion cannot be visualized entirely (unsatisfactory colposcopy). The procedure is done to rule out occult invasive disease.

A. A biopsy is positive for CIN III. Excision of the transformation zone is required (cone biopsy).

B. Even if the repeat ECC is negative, there is still the indication for cervical conization with the CIN biopsy result.

C. See answer to A.

E. The purpose of the cervical conization is to rule out an occult malignancy. If a hysterectomy is done, and an invasive carcinoma is found, then the wrong procedure may have been done, and the patient's final prognosis may be worse.

ANSWER 90

A. It is important to remember that a Pap smear is only a screening test for cervical cancer. If a Pap smear is done of a visible cancer, it will only show cancer about 50% of the time. With a visible lesion, you must biopsy the lesion to diagnose; if it is invasive cancer then you would proceed with the appropriate staging workup. If the biopsy came back as microinvasive, a cone biopsy would be the next step.

B. Although this could be a herpetic lesion, any visible lesion of the cervix must be biopsied to rule out malignancy.

C. A Pap smear is only a screen. In the face of a visible cancerous lesion, the Pap smear will not be conclusive for cancer in a significant percentage of cases. If a lesion is seen, a biopsy must be done.

D. Although this could be a primary syphilitic chancre, the most likely diagnosis is a cervical neoplasia.

E. This would be done if the biopsy came back inconclusive for invasion (i.e., microinvasive). If the punch biopsy came back conclusive for a frankly invasive carcinoma, it would be at least a stage IB, requiring radical hysterectomy or radiation therapy.

ANSWER 91

E. The Pap smear is a screening test. Although the cervix appears normal to the naked eye, once acetic acid is applied and the magnification of the colposcope added, vascular abnormalities will often be seen. The most concerning colposcopic finding is the presence of abnormal vessels. These suggest carcinoma *in situ* or invasive carcinoma. If the colposcopic exam is negative, a cone biopsy is performed to find the source of the suspicious cells.

A. This is the therapy for early stage cervical carcinoma. The diagnosis of cancer has not yet been made. A biopsy is necessary.

B. Simple hysterectomy is not the proper cure for invasive cervical carcinoma. Also, the diagnosis of cancer has not yet been made. A biopsy is necessary.

C. It is still likely that a cone biopsy will be necessary if a colposcopic exam is unsatisfactory. The first step, however, in the workup, is a colposcopy with directed biopsy. If invasive cancer is then found, appropriate therapy can be started.

D. Cryotherapy is only indicated for low-grade dysplastic lesions of the cervix, after adequate colposcopic exam to rule out malignancy.

ANSWER 92

B. Adnexal masses can be found in all age groups, though there are differences in the prevalence of certain conditions based on the patient's age. After menopause, the ovaries become nonpalpable, so any enlargement should make one suspicious for cancer. In the reproductive age, functional cysts are common. These can be up to 6 cm or more, so any simple cyst less than 6 cm can be observed for several cycles. If still present, a workup is indicated.

A. Various etiologies for adnexal masses have different incidences depending on the patient's age. Germ cell neoplasms are more likely to be found in younger women. Ectopics will be found only in reproductive age women. Epithelial malignancies are more common in postmenopausal women.

C. See answer to A.

D. Any palpable ovary in a postmenopausal woman needs to be evaluated to rule out a malignancy.

E. Any solid mass of the ovary needs to be evaluated to rule out a malignancy.

ANSWER 93

C. In a postmenopausal woman, the ovaries should not be palpable; if they are, it should raise the concern that an ovarian malignancy is present. Before one would perform an operative evaluation, radiologic assessment should be done.

A. Although this is an accepted regimen for estrogen replacement therapy, the palpable ovaries need to be evaluated to rule out malignancy.

B. Although this is an accepted regimen for estrogen replacement therapy, the palpable ovaries need to be evaluated to rule out malignancy.

D. Dual photon densitometry will give a reliable measure of bone density. Again, however, the palpable ovary is the first thing that needs to be worked up.

E. Although surgical exploration may be warranted, initial workup of the adnexal mass should include an ultrasound along with tumor markers. A CT scan may also be warranted.

ANSWER 94

C. DES exposure is associated with adenosis and clear cell adenocarcinoma of the vagina and cervix. If a patient is nulliparous, obese, and reaches menopause at age 52 or later, there appears to be a 5-fold increase in the risk of endometrial cancer over the patient who does not fulfill these criteria. Also upper body fat localization, which is related to lower serum hormone-bound globulin and higher endogenous production of nonprotein-bound estradiol, is a risk factor for endometrial cancer.

A. Increased relative risk for developing endometrial adenocarcinoma.

B. Increased relative risk for developing endometrial adenocarcinoma.

D. Increased relative risk for developing endometrial adenocarcinoma due to an increase in the circulating levels of estrogens (peripheral conversion of androgens to estrogens by the adipose tissue).

E. Increased relative risk for developing endometrial adenocarcinoma due to the long exposure to unopposed estrogen.

ANSWER 95

A. In a virginal 7-year-old, the best way to examine a lower abdominal process is with a rectal examination, not with a vaginal exam. Rectal exam will be able to detect most pelvic and lower abdominal masses.

B. Vaginal exam in a 7-year-old should be avoided.

C. See answer to B.

D. A lower abdominal may be missed by percussion, unless it is large enough to have a significant portion within the abdominal cavity.

ANSWER 96

C. During intercourse, the vagina can significantly expand and elongate. After surgical reconstruction of the vagina or with creation of a neovagina, intercourse is the best technique to maintain normal caliber and size of the vagina when compared with dilators.

A. Dilation of the hymen is unnecessary.

B. With a normal exam, explanation of the normal physiology of the female sexual response is the appropriate next step.

D. No surgical procedures are indicated.

E. See above explanation.

ANSWER 97

C. Beneficence is the obligation to promote the well being of others. Justice is the right of individuals to claim what is due them based on certain personal properties or characteristics. Informed consent can be defined as the willing acceptance of a medical intervention after adequate disclosure by the physician. Honesty means that the patient is given complete and truthful information about her condition. Confidentiality means that a patient has the right to make decisions about her own care and to decide to whom these decisions and her medical information are communicated.

A. Honesty means that the patient is given complete and truthful information about her condition.

B. Beneficence is the obligation to promote the well being of others.

D. Informed consent can be defined as the willing acceptance of a medical intervention after adequate disclosure by the physician.

E. Justice is the right of individuals to claim what is due them based on certain personal properties or characteristics.

ANSWER 98

A. Part of the normal aging process changes in the human sexual response. Although it is natural for a 66-year-old man to take longer to achieve an erection, it is possible that other factors may be involved. This includes the use of other medications and chronic medical conditions. Should this be the case, then appropriate referral is indicated.

B. See above explanation.

C. See above explanation.

D. See above explanation.

E. See above explanation.

ANSWER 99

D. Again, this covers the ethical concept of confidentiality. Even though her husband is the father of the affected child, the patient has the right to request that you do not disclose this information to him.

A. See above discussion.

B. See above discussion.

C. See above discussion.

E. See above discussion.

ANSWER 100

B. A helpful technique when examining any young child is to place the child's hand on top of the physician's hand during the abdominal exam. This can help divert the child's attention if she is ticklish and give the child a sense of control.

A. Diversion attempts are often unsuccessful with a ticklish child.

C. Applying increased pressure may only make the exam more painful to the patient and thus more difficult.

D. Restraining the child by anyone will make the exam much more difficult and potentially more traumatic to the child.

E. Restraining the child by anyone will make the exam much more difficult and potentially more traumatic to the child.